Health On Fire

In the name of the highest wisdom who governs the whole universe

Health On Fire

Restore Your Ultimate Health Today!

The Raw Living Path to Detox, Natural Healing And Lifelong Vitality

Michael Zara

"Amidst the ebb and flow of daily life, there exists a silent sentinel, guarding the fortress of our well-being with unwavering dedication."

"To your Ultimate Health"

Health on Fire – Restore Your Ultimate Health Today

First Published in Australia in 2024

©Michael Zara 2024

For consent contact: info@michaelzara.com.au

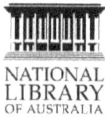

NATIONAL LIBRARY OF AUSTRALIA

A catalogue record for this book is available from the National Library of Australia

ISBN: **978-1-7637322-0-9**

Michael Zara acknowledges the Traditional Custodians of the lands upon which we live and work and pays respect to elders past and present.

Michael Zara proudly supports and sponsors the charities below:

- National Breast Cancer Foundation- Australia
- Vipassana Meditation Cantres- Australia

To my beloved wife **Emma**, who has always supported me and my wonderful children **Ryan**, **Leo**, and **Ava**, whom my heart always goes with.

Foreword

"Zara's passion is infectious... The book stirred something in me. It's rare that a health book pushes me this hard to question my habits and look closely at what I put in my body every day."

Health on Fire is a fiery manifesto about reclaiming health through radical changes in diet and lifestyle. Michael Zara lays out his philosophy of "Ultimate Health," arguing that many of our modern health issues come not from aging, genetics, or bad luck, but from what and how we eat, especially our reliance on cooked and processed foods. Through personal stories, analogies, and a strong critique of mainstream medicine and food culture, Zara builds his case for a raw vegan lifestyle, one stripped of salt, oil, cooking, and even many widely accepted beliefs about nutrition. At its core, the book aims to help readers wake up from passive conformity and take ownership of their physical and emotional wellbeing.

Zara's passion is infectious. He clearly cares deeply about helping people feel better, and his personal transformation adds credibility to his message. I appreciated his effort to explain complicated concepts like oxidation, immune function, and enzyme loss in plain language. Some of the metaphors, like the frog in boiling water or the apple turning brown, landed powerfully. They made me think differently about what I eat and what I consider "normal." Zara's strong stance against cooked food and his deep passion for raw eating at times felt more rooted in personal philosophy. While some critiques of mainstream health systems may feel bold or unconventional, they are clearly rooted in deep conviction and **lived experience**.

One of the strongest aspects is the book's clear and logical structure. Each chapter builds smoothly on the last, guiding the reader from foundational ideas into more complex topics. Zara takes care to ground his advice in basic biological principles, such as metabolism, oxidation, and enzyme function, and explains them in simple, straightforward language. The book is written in a way that's approachable and engaging, with plenty of relatable examples. Best of all, it gives real, actionable steps. Whether it's shifting toward raw foods or rethinking hydration and sleep, there's always something practical to try.

The book stirred something in me. It's rare that a health book pushes me this hard to question my habits and look closely at what I put in my body every day. I've already started paying more attention to raw foods and how I feel after different meals. Zara's diet recommendations are quite focused and may be challenging. While his approach is clearly shaped by personal transformation and deep conviction, the book leans more on lived experience. This gives his message a sincere and **passionate tone**.

Health on Fire is for readers who are ready to challenge the status quo. If you're tired of feeling tired, open to radical change, and don't mind a blunt voice with strong opinions, you'll probably come away from this book fired up. This book will stick with you. Zara doesn't just want you to read it, he wants you to wake up.

Thomas Anderson

Literary Titan

This **transformative book** is a manifesto for reclaiming health through the healing power of raw, living foods. Drawing on over two decades of research and personal healing, Michael Zara challenges conventional health beliefs and delivers an evidence-based path to naturally reversing and managing chronic conditions.

What makes *Health on Fire* stand out is its clarity and honesty in a world flooded with health misinformation. Written in simple, actionable language, it empowers readers with truths that many have never been told; offering not just knowledge, but practical steps to reclaim vitality and live fully. Bold, eye-opening, and deeply empowering, this book is already changing lives.

Authors Book Launch & Expo (ABLE Group)

Preface

May all have a world free of all diseases and complications, full of love and peace.

Before starting, I would like to declare:

As an educated person, I've always honored science and technology. I believe it is part of our soul advancement; medical and agricultural science are no exceptions.

Doctors, nurses, medical workers, and medical scientists have contributed significantly to our lives and the well-being of humans on Earth. This is the same for the agricultural industry.

I always respect doctors; they do wonderful jobs, particularly in emergencies, accidents, and pregnancy complications.

"A healthy person has a thousand dreams. A sick person may only have one!"

This book aims to help people be free of diseases and live with Ultimate Health at the highest possible energy level. What is Ultimate Health? Let us discuss it in detail, but first, a disclaimer.

Disclaimer

The information in the book is being collected, investigated, and shared in the best faith by the Author. The information provided in this book is solely for informational purposes and comes without any assurance of absolute accuracy. It is not intended to be construed as medical advice.

This book is written as general advice based on the Author's experience. The Author and publisher disclaim any responsibility for any health complications that may arise from following the advice presented in this book. Under no circumstances shall the Author have any liability to you for reliance on the information published in this book.

Anyone (including you) is responsible for their health and must do their due diligence and assess any risks associated with changing their lifestyle and diet. They must seek advice from their health practitioner or medical advisor before deciding to follow alternative lifestyles and diets, especially the ones suggested in this book.

A Quick Note Before We Begin

Thank you for picking up *Health on Fire*. I wrote this book to help you reconnect with your body's natural design and take control of your health, from the inside out.

As you read, if you find value in these insights or feel inspired to make changes in your life, I'd be deeply grateful if you'd consider leaving a review when you're done. I put the links at the end of the book.

It's a small gesture that helps this message reach more people who are searching for real answers.

Wishing you clarity, strength, and health,
— **Michael Zara**

Contents

Chapter 1

A Health Story

Imagine one day your family doctor calls you and says: "Hey, I haven't seen you for ages, have you changed your GP[1]?

You respond:

"No, I haven't. I only changed my lifestyle and eating habits... and now I've discovered my Ultimate Health!"

They paused, surprised:

"Seriously? If this is true, let's catch up for a coffee, I want to know your secret."

What if you could meet your doctor not just for a routine checkup, but to share your health story, a life lived naturally, fully, and free from disease? Many people accept that being sick is normal. They believe a cold, headaches, or fatigue are just part of life. And when they don't feel well, they grab a painkiller or throat lozenge without a second thought.

But what if you could live differently? What if your body already knows how to heal, and all you need to do is stop getting in its way?

Picture this: You wake up tomorrow feeling different. No snooze button, no dragging yourself out of bed. Your skin feels fresh.

---

[1] A GP or a General Practitioner is a doctor who is also qualified in general medical practice.

Your mind is alert. You glance in the mirror and see a spark in your eyes you haven't noticed in years.

Sounds impossible? I thought so too.

I wasn't born with perfect health. For years, I followed what experts told me: the food pyramid, the latest "superfoods," even trendy diets promising miracles. But my body had other plans. Cracks started small, an ache here, an itch there. Then the list grew: severe migraines, high fever, infections, skin rashes, fatigue, brain fog, digestive troubles and later high blood pressure. Doctors ran tests. The results came back "normal." Prescriptions, creams, vague advice like "reduce stress" or "eat more balanced meals" ... but nothing changed- except my frustration.

I remember looking at my reflection one morning, my skin inflamed, my eyes dull, and thinking: *Is this really it? Is this how it's going to be from now on?*

Then came the turning point, not in a hospital, nor in a clinic, but in the most unexpected way. I stumbled on something that seemed too simple to work, yet too consistent to ignore. At first, I resisted. It went against almost everything I had been taught. But desperation has a way of breaking disbelief. So, I tried it.

The changes weren't overnight, but they were undeniable. Within days, my energy returned. Weeks later, my skin cleared. Months later, I was living in a body that felt ten years younger, without expensive supplements, without starving myself, without extreme fads.

What I discovered isn't a trend. It isn't magic. It's the way human bodies are designed to thrive. You already have the ability to heal, but modern living has buried it under layers of habits, misinformation, and damage.

By the end of this book, you'll see food, health, and your body in a completely different light. Some of what you read might challenge everything you've believed, but if you keep an open mind, you'll discover how to:

• Reverse chronic symptoms

• Tap into natural, steady energy

• Restore balance without relying on pills or endless doctor visits

Your body is waiting. The question is: are you ready to **set your health on fire**?

Before we go further, I have one request: please set aside whatever you have heard about disease, food, nutrition, and diet until you finish this book. Read with an open mind, free of prejudice or preconceived ideas. Much of what you'll discover here may be brand new; and to truly understand it, you'll need curiosity more than certainty. What you're about to read may even challenge what you've always believed to be "normal."

My own journey is about rediscovering health, yet the reality is that many people's lives follow a very different path. To show you what I mean, let me share a story that might sound familiar.

Meet Tom; a boy who grew up on a farm far from the city. Tom is energetic and healthy and participates in many daily activities. His parents consider their lifestyle to be a healthy one. They usually provide Tom with food recommended by society and the government, based on the standard food pyramid. This includes bread, cereal, rice, pasta, and potatoes; some fruits and vegetables;

meat, poultry, dairy, eggs, fish; and finally, some sweets like chocolate and cakes[1].

Living away from the city, they rarely dine out during the week and avoid junk food. Since they have their own farm, many of their food ingredients come from high-quality natural sources. There is little water contamination and air pollution, and they are mostly away from technologies, which minimises distractions and stress.

Wow! What a wonderful lifestyle, including a natural and ideal diet. Based on our shared beliefs, our little Tom lives a healthy life full of energy, free from complications and diseases. Imagine living in such conditions; what an ideal life that would be! Wouldn't it?

But wait a minute, let's look closer at what our little Tom's life really looks like. He occasionally gets headaches, catches colds regularly during winter, and suffers from hay fever with lots of sneezes and coughing in spring. Some days, he deals with an upset stomach, which keeps him in the toilet more than usual.

These all seem natural for a young boy, right? No worries, who cares? His parents help him with medication for every situation, from Panadol[2] for his fevers to antihistamines[3] for allergies, providing him with some relief from pain and discomfort. He also has mild asthma, and his parents have been told that asthma is common in many kids, and he only needs to take a steroid spray to relieve it.

He grows older, becomes a teenager, goes to university, graduates, and eventually becomes an adult who decides to be a farmer like

---

[1] I would call it the Typical Western Diet (T.W.D.) which comprises fresh and cooked food. (see Glossary)

[2] Panadol is a brand name for the drug paracetamol, which is also known as acetaminophen in some countries.

[3] Antihistamines are a class of drugs that counteract the effects of histamine (see Glossary)

his father. He marries a wonderful young lady who has a similar lifestyle to what she learned from her *parents and society*. They continue the same lifestyle as their parents, with subtle changes due to the new materials available on the market.

But Tom gradually notices that his energy is not at the same level it was when he was a boy. He becomes sick more often, needs more medication, and sometimes spends longer periods in the toilet. Over the years, he also notices more frequent headaches, higher blood pressure, elevated bad blood cholesterol levels, and Type 2 diabetes[1]. His skin is not as soft and flexible as it used to be. Like many others, he regularly takes various medications based on health advice to manage his condition and keep his health complications under control.

He also remembers that his parents had some of these issues. He was told that these things happen to many people as they get older.

His health advisor confirms that genes play a key role: "While we inherit our genes from our parents, most of these health issues come from them." (It is easy to blame the genes, isn't it?)

Tom notices that one of his particularly severe health issues is migraines, but neither of his parents nor any of his siblings had them. He was asked to search around and see if any uncles or aunties had migraines; again, the answer was no. What about in-laws? Did any of them or even their neighbors have the same or similar severe headaches? (Trying to find the genes and blame them!)

---

[1] Type 2 diabetes is a chronic condition that affects the way the body processes blood sugar (glucose). (see Glossary)

Years later, our friend Tom is now old enough with grandkids who are about to graduate from university. They need to push Tom's wheelchair to attend their graduation ceremonies.

Tom's wheelchair also has a side bag filled with a full spectrum of pills and tablets, plus a couple of different bottles of medicines to manage his newly added health issues such as Parkinson's[1], memory loss, thrombophilia[2], and lastly, ALS[3]. He thinks about how his medical needs have evolved from a couple of painkillers per week to a bag of fifty-plus tablets, and even some nappies!

But he believes he is lucky not to have developed serious illnesses such as cancer or cardiovascular disease, which killed several of his friends and his beloved wife.

Does Tom's story sound familiar? I hope you aren't like Tom, but you might know someone like him. What about your parents? Grandparents? Uncles, aunts, or even one of your neighbors?

How often have you heard from health advisors or the media that many health complications for adults, the elderly, and even children are normal? Or that most of these issues are genetic and therefore normal? Have you ever looked back at what your parents were doing and realised *how you simply copied them*?

I thought about this for years and years. Often, taking responsibility can be challenging, especially regarding our health and lifestyle. We do our best to follow the standards dictated by society and leave the responsibility to the government, health organisations, our health practitioners, and even **our parents**.

---

[1] A nerve disease which affects movements. (see Glossary)

[2] A tendency of the blood to form clots. (see Glossary)

[3] ALS stands for Amyotrophic Lateral Sclerosis, also known as Lou Gehrig's disease. (see Glossary)

The biggest problem is that almost everyone; young or old, no matter their profession, has some health issues. Even scientists, doctors, and government officials often rely on medications, which makes illness seem "normal." It's much like a child growing up in a home where both parents smoke: to them, smoking feels like a natural part of life.

It doesn't have to be this way. Change is the key! If anyone decides to change their lifestyle and address the real needs of their body appropriately, they may achieve their Ultimate Health. But what is Ultimate Health?

The Ultimate Health

Now, considering all the above, I would like to define 'Ultimate Health'.

Ultimate Health means having a healthy body, being full of energy, and being free from diseases and most medications. I say 'most' because you may still need medication for some occasions, depending on the damage done to your body. Some medications might also help the body return to a healthy state more quickly.

You may have heard that achieving this requires a lifestyle that includes a proper diet (food and drink), clean air, good mental health, and regular physical exercise. There are three simple steps you need to take:

1. Understand your body functions and its nutrition requirements
2. Give your body and mind the proper fuel
3. Maintain your Ultimate Health by a natural lifestyle

The natural lifestyle we are going to explore in this book is not the one being advertised or accepted by a society dependent on medications. It is a lifestyle where your body parts work at their optimum performance, all organs are relaxed and receive the best nutrition and energy, your mind is at peace, and you feel great all the time, all day, and all year round, regardless of your age.

The above statement may seem ambiguous, and you might wonder if I am dreaming. Yes, I am dreaming, but this dream can soon become your reality. To achieve Ultimate Health, several essential elements must come together. I would categorise them into four parts:

1- Diet and body-feeding lifestyle

2- Daily physical activity and exercise

3- Deep Sleep

4- Relaxed mind

Although we will cover all four parts, our primary focus will be on the first part, as it greatly influences and supports the other three. With a healthy physical body, you can exercise regularly, sleep deeply, and maintain a relaxed mind. Together, these elements can bring you the Ultimate Health we all dream of.

Now, let's take a closer look at how we nourish the physical body, because the truth is, most diseases don't come from bad luck or genetics, but from what we put on our plates every single day. The foods we eat either strengthen our body's natural defence and repair systems, or they slowly damage and overwhelm them, leading to sickness. A natural lifestyle isn't just helpful; it is essential for lasting **health and happiness**.

Capture 2

Why Eating?

I have a question: what is the main reason for eating?

I raised this question several times in my meetings and talks and received various answers.

"Because I get hungry!"

"To fill my stomach!"

"We need food to be alive!"

And some people said they "love eating"

Enjoying, addressing hunger, and filling the stomach can all be correct.

Eating is one of the basic human needs. According to science, we eat primarily for two reasons: **energy** and **nutrition**. We require energy to function, and nutrition is essential for cell renewal and the maintenance of bodily functions, including cells reproduction.

Humans consume a variety of foods prepared in numerous ways. Some foods, such as fruits and certain vegetables, are eaten raw. Others are cooked using various methods, including boiling, steaming, stir-frying, and even deep frying.

While we may use a combination of these methods, heating changes the natural structure of food and reduces its nutritional value. Over time, this affects how well our cells are nourished when we eat cooked food. Let's see how this happens.

Creating Energy

Science tells us that one of the main reasons for eating is to create energy.

Every machine requires energy to be operational, and our bodies are no exception. People may think we only need energy to work, walk, or run. In fact, we need energy for every single moment of our lives. Even when we are resting or sleeping, our organs require energy to perform their functions.

Energy can be produced in many ways, such as hydraulic, kinetic, or nuclear. One fundamental way to create energy is by burning materials. For example, burning wood produces heat, a type of energy. Our intelligent body uses a similar process to produce energy, known as metabolism.

In simple terms, burning occurs when a material mixes with oxygen; this process is called oxidation in chemistry. When firewood mixes with oxygen, a fire occurs, generating heat as a form of energy.

We eat food and inhale oxygen. With the help of catalysts, these two mix inside our body cells. The food material gets oxidised (burnt) and creates energy.

In chemistry, oxidation can occur more rapidly due to two key factors: first, moisture; and second, heat. The higher the moisture content and temperature, the faster materials oxidise.

Have you ever seen a piece of steel or iron rust when exposed to moisture? That rusting is simply oxidation. We protect metal with coatings, such as paint, to slow down this process.

You can conduct a simple test yourself: apply heat to a piece of bare steel, expose it to moisture and oxygen, and observe how quickly it rusts (oxidises).

On another note, nearly every material has an outer protective layer to shield it from oxidation. This is because oxygen is highly reactive and constantly seeks out raw materials to combine with. Its high electronegativity indicates how strongly it can attract electrons from other substances.

Have you ever noticed that many fruits have a hard outer layer? What happens if you remove this outer layer and leave the fruit exposed to the environment? For example, apples have a hard skin that serves to protect the inner fruit. If you peel off the skin and leave the apple exposed to the air, the inner part will begin to change color and darken. The same happens to a banana if you peel it and expose it to oxygen.

This is the oxidising process; over time, you'll likely observe changes in color and taste, often resulting in a rancid or spoiled state. And here's something to think about: do we really want to consume the parts of food that have already been exposed to oxygen?

Now, let's consider what happens when we cook our food. We break the protective layer of the food ingredients by cutting, chopping, or grinding. Then, we put them in a pot and heat them with the addition of water or presentation of moisture.

Cooking essentially means:

1. Removing the protective layer of most raw materials
2. Heat the raw materials
3. Exposing them to water or in the presence of moisture

By completing these three steps, what are we doing? The answer is we are forcing the ingredients to oxidise more rapidly. The higher the temperature, the more components break down and oxidise.

Here's the problem: if something is already oxidised, our body cannot extract the same level of energy from it again. The efficiency is lost. You may ask: how do people who eat mostly cooked food still survive and have energy?

The answer is that not all of the inner cells are oxidised during cooking; some survive the process. Most people also eat some fresh fruits, vegetables, or salads, and even unhealthy foods like fast-food burgers usually contain a slice of tomato or lettuce. The fact is, the amount of energy we can get from cooked food, which is already partially oxidised, is far less compared to fully raw food. Raw parts such as tomato and lettuce still keep their enzymes and vitamins, which support metabolism and help maintain some level of energy in people following a standard diet (T.W.D.[1]).

To clarify it further, the energy produced by burning a piece of wood is **much higher** than that produced by burning the same amount of charcoal. Why? Because charcoal is already *partially oxidised and burnt.*

Living exclusively on cooked food could pose serious risks over time, because essential nutrients and energy potential are lost during the cooking process. I couldn't find definitive scientific research specifically on the effects of feeding humans or laboratory mice exclusively cooked food.

However, I did the experiment myself. For one week, I ate only cooked food, with no fresh vegetables or fruits. The result? By the

---

[1] Typical Western Diet- which is widely accepted by many people in Europe, America, and Australia as a food pyramid and model for human nutrition. This food pyramid, which includes cooked foods, is also accepted by many people around the globe.

end of day seven, my energy was completely drained. It was one of the most unpleasant experiences I've had with food.

If you're curious, you don't need to repeat my exact test; but try noticing how your body feels when you increase or decrease the amount of raw food in your diet. Many people are surprised at the difference in their energy.

If you do experiment with this, I'd love to hear about your experience on my website: www.michaelzara.com

.

Nutrition

I mentioned that our body needs nutrition for bodily functions, to support metabolism with catalysts, and to reproduce cells.

According to science, our bodies require nutrients from five main groups:

1- Carbohydrates

2- Proteins (built from amino acids)

3- Vitamins

4- Minerals

5- Lipids (fats)

We should consume almost all these nutrients daily for optimal health.

While you may consume raw food, cooked food prepared using various methods is often favored. Heating raw materials through cooking alters the nature of most ingredients and generates new ones. Let's explore this transformation process.

Imagine we have boiling water in a pot, and someone puts their hand in it for 1 minute. What happens to the hand when it's removed? Now, what if the hand were kept in the boiling pot for half an hour? What would its shape be then? Do you think hot water burns?

We do the same thing to our food ingredients by heating them. In deep frying, instead of 100°C, we heat the ingredients to 250°C. The higher the temperature, the greater the damage to food's natural structure.

What we call cooking is, in truth, a kind of controlled burning!

Nature already prepares raw foods for us; ripened under the sun, they come ready to nourish us without needing further heating (or burning).

The truth is that during cooking (or burning), the natural structure of the ingredients is mostly destroyed, creating new burnt and oxidised substances. During cooking (or burning), all enzymes are lost, and most vitamins, as well as some live minerals (particularly trace elements), are destroyed.

For example, Vitamin C is highly susceptible to destruction by heat. While Vitamin E is more heat-resistant, prolonged exposure can still lead to its degradation. Additionally, minerals can oxidise during the cooking process, making them less effective for our bodies to process and absorb.

According to research (see References) heating raw materials creates free radicals, and you may have heard that antioxidants are required to neutralise them. Vitamin C and Vitamin E are the best-known antioxidants we need daily. But they can lose their antioxidant property when heated and may even become pro-oxidants. Pro-oxidants are agents that promote the production of reactive oxygen species, and free radicals, what an irony!

Do you always use oil when cooking? Even if you grill your food (a so-called healthier way of cooking), fatty acids (oil) are still present in the ingredients, especially in meat. Heating the lipids (fats) will create lipid peroxidation, a very reactive free radical; by consuming them, your body can experience oxidative stress (see References).

This happens to proteins as well. Proteins containing amino acids such as methionine, cysteine, arginine, and histidine are the most vulnerable to oxidation. Oxidatively damaged protein products often contain highly reactive groups that can contribute to damaging cell membranes and DNA.

As you have observed, oxidised materials lose much of their nutritional value and can even contribute to toxicity in our bodies. The purpose of eating food that has been burnt (so-called 'cooked') is compromised. We don't derive the same quality of energy from oxidised foods, because their nature has been changed.

If you remember the earlier example of peeled bananas and apples exposed to oxygen, no one willingly eats the inner part of a fruit that has been left out in the open, exposed to air, heat, and gone spoiled. Because we believe they are harmful and dangerous and generally, do not taste good. Yet at the same time, we accept foods exposed to air, moisture, and heat; partly burnt by high temperatures, and still consider them **healthy**. *Isn't that striking?*

Capture 3

Cooking Paradigm

You may love cooking, enjoy eating cooked food, and watching cooking shows like MasterChef[1]. But have you ever asked yourself why we need to cook our food? What is the main reason for using hot plates and applying heat to raw materials in pots or pans?

When asking these questions, one main answer often emerges: everyone cooks. Even intelligent individuals and leaders such as professors, politicians, doctors, and health scientists engage in cooking. If cooking were problematic, why would so many intelligent humans keep doing it without questioning the potential downsides?

We heat, fry, grill, and roast almost everything: as if raw food needed a makeover before being worthy of our plates.

Let us think about it briefly and see why we insist on heating (or as I sometimes call it, "burning") our food.

Created Paradox

You might be familiar with our habit paradoxes and their origins. Here I'll share some of them.

---

[1] "MasterChef" is a popular competitive cooking reality television show that has been adapted in numerous countries around the world.

Years ago, an experiment was conducted using a group of monkeys, placing them in a cage. Inside the cage was a ladder leading to a platform in the middle, with some bananas placed on top.

When one monkey spotted the bananas, it began climbing the ladder to reach the fresh fruit.

The scientists conducting the experiment had installed shower heads above the cage. When the monkey climbed the ladder, they activated a very cold and icy water shower, soaking the monkey on top. This cold-water punishment effectively discouraged the monkey from climbing, and the scientists stopped it once the monkey descended.

The process was repeated with the next monkey, using the cold shower as punishment once again. This continued until all the monkeys in the cage refrained from attempting to climb the ladder. Over a few days, none of them tried to reach the bananas because of their fear of the icy-water punishment.

Later, a new monkey was introduced to the cage. Upon seeing the tempting bananas, this recent addition instinctively began climbing the ladder. However, the other monkeys, who had learned to avoid the cold water, immediately pounced on the new monkey, pulling it down and scaring it away from the ladder.

The confused new monkey eventually surrendered, as the others refused to let it climb again. Scientists repeated the pattern by replacing another original monkey with a new one. As soon as the new monkey started to climb, the others would pull it down and punch it.

In the end, all the original monkeys were gradually replaced with new ones, one by one, and none of the monkeys tried to climb the ladder to pick a banana. Interestingly, even though none of the new monkeys had ever experienced the cold-water punishment, they still refrained from climbing the ladder because of the learned behavior of the original group.

Isn't that fascinating? It shows how behaviour can outlive its original reason.

Now, you might think: "Well, animals don't have our level of intelligence; surely humans would do better." But do we?

Let's observe how we behave in similar situations, using human examples.

Social Conformity

A social experiment was conducted by National Geographic under the series called "Brain Games" couple of years ago, and I watched it on YouTube.

The experiment was terrific, watching how humans act in similar situations. The aim was to investigate whether each person acts the same way as others or whether we use our brains to decide differently. Let me explain what I observed.

A large room was arranged for the experiment, with all the actors seated on chairs, patiently awaiting their turn for an eye examination. Then, a lady in a purple dress entered the room for her eye exam, completely unaware of the experiment or the authenticity of the other participants.

She was surprised when everyone stood up as soon as they heard a beep. She hesitated and didn't stand up until the third beep, feeling embarrassed as she looked at the others. However, the third beep worked, and she began mimicking the others by standing up with each subsequent beep.

After all the actors were removed from the room one by one and had visited the eye examiner, the lady in the purple dress continued to stand up at every beep and sit down soon after, despite being alone in the room. Fascinating, isn't it?

But the most remarkable part came next. A man entered and began reading a magazine. When the lady in the purple dress stood up, he asked her why. She then instructed him to do the same. And guess what? He followed suit, standing and sitting at every beep!

Subsequently, more people entered the room and began doing the same, without knowing the reason behind this strange behavior.

I was as surprised as you probably are now: how easily others' actions can influence individuals, even without a rational basis. It challenges the notion of our uniqueness and highlights our **tendency to conform** to group behavior.

I recommend watching it on YouTube a couple of times and thinking about the behaviors we often follow without questioning why.

I watched another example on YouTube. A test conducted on people when they joined a group of actors in a lift. The actors, all doing the same odd thing, faced the back of the lift. And sure enough, strangers soon turned around too, following the group and mimicking the behaviour, even though it made no sense.

Social conformity is defined as a specific type of influence that results in a change of behaviour or belief to fit in with a group. People tend to unquestioningly follow the crowd, especially with repeated actions. This is not usually harmful; as social beings, adopting the behaviour of a crowd can help humans survive in many challenging situations and threats to our race, such as during wars and *natural disasters*.

However, in some cases, it causes issues when the reason behind the crowd's actions no longer exists, yet we continue to react in the same way as before. On the other hand, the desire to be accepted can be harmful. For example, young individuals may start smoking to gain acceptance from a new group of smoker friends. They desire conformity and dislike feeling like a stranger.

The web has more examples. If you are interested in learning more, do your research, especially read and watch the examples about social conformity.

Now you can see how a paradox happens: most of us never stop to ask why we apply heat to our food. Someone started this hundreds of thousands of years ago when humans discovered fire, and since then the habit has continued; rarely questioned.

I raised this question several times and have yet to get a logical answer.

Most of the responses I received felt more like traditions or assumptions than genuine scientific explanations. It would be wonderful if you could ask this question many times to yourself and others. I would love to hear the answers.

Several individuals offered a response to this query. Some voiced concerns over eating raw meats. Throughout the upcoming chapters, I will delve into whether humans are naturally inclined to be meat eaters. But before we continue, may I ask why you cook your vegetables?

These days people even heat-treat some of their fruits! Yes, people bake bananas or pineapples; as if nature hadn't done a good enough job already. Heating, frying, or baking almost everything has become the norm, even though we rarely stop to question what cooking actually does to our food."

Although some research suggests that cooking can make certain nutrients more bioavailable, for example lycopene in tomatoes and beta-carotene in carrots, what about the vanishing vitamin C, enzymes, and other delicate nutrients that are damaged or destroyed by heat? Even this small improvement does not happen in most food ingredients.

Gradual Harm

You may think we eat cooked food, and it does not harm or hurt. You may overlook the harm when it gradually happens.

Let me share another experiment.

If you put a frog in hot water, it will jump out in a second! However, if you put it in a bowl full of water at room temperature and gradually warm the water until it gets really hot, the frog stays there until it dies! Its reaction to a gradual heat is nothing, whilst it reacts quickly to a sudden change.

Humans are not different from that frog. We react to a **sudden change** quickly; but we can handle gradual changes with faith!

If you go to a supermarket and suddenly notice that the price of a product has doubled, you will likely have a strong reaction. However, if it increases by just a couple of cents, you may not even notice it.

The same is valid for changing seasons; snow in the middle of summer is such a surprise, while there is no surprise when the temperature gradually drops until it gets to winter with snowfalls.

Another example is a smoker. I've seen heavy smokers who have been living and smoking for over 30 years.

First-time smokers experience severe vertigo, making it impossible to stand. I tested, and I almost fainted. However, after a couple of weeks of smoking, the cigarette may no longer have any noticeable effect on the person, even if they smoke a full pack a day! What has happened here? Do cigarettes affect them? Of course, it does. Their body gradually starts adapting itself to the toxins introduced by smoking, and sometimes, it doesn't have the same effect.

This is the gradual harm that we may not notice at all. How might we describe the life of a heavy smoker? Does their body get hurt? What will happen when they quit, and can they get back to a natural life without smoking? I leave these questions for you to answer.

You see what we are doing by putting toxins in our bodies. There are similarities between the toxins from smoke and from heat-treated food. Although not identical, both place a heavy burden on the body over time. Consuming cooked food over a long period can have a detrimental effect on our health, with noticeable consequences emerging later in life, particularly as we reach middle age.

When a baby is born, they do not consume cooked food. However, as they grow, they are gradually introduced to toxins, and their bodies adapt to them. This gradual exposure can lead to harm that may go unnoticed. A lot of babies have a strong reaction to cooked food by vomiting or diarrhea.

Even at a very young age, you may consider it natural to have pain in your stomach after each meal. Many even consider it normal to suffer constipation, or to undergo surgeries later in life for conditions that have built up gradually. It is common for harm to go unnoticed until it becomes incurable, often because of its gradual progression. Remember the frog in hot water, and you can imagine the condition of a person with a terminal illness.

Once you cleanse your body using appropriate, natural raw foods, you'll notice a swift and noticeable reaction if you reintroduce toxins through cooked food. In many cases, individuals with a natural lifestyle and a clean body may find it challenging to tolerate oxidised materials. If you have a clean body and try heat treated (special deep fried food like French fries), you might become aware of the toxins you introduced to your body in the past and their harmful effects.

I had always considered wholemeal bread one of my healthiest foods. However, after 18 months of following my natural, fully Raw Vegan lifestyle, I decided to test it by eating a piece of bread.

I was shocked at how my body reacted to this cooked food! Almost immediately, I developed a light headache and stomach pain, and it took some time to eliminate it from my digestive system.

The experiment showed me that gradual harm is deceptive; perhaps we are not as far from that **poor frog** in a boiling pot as we might like to think!

Tasty Foods

One answer I got from my interviews when I asked my popular question about why we need to cook our food was: "We love our cooked foods because they are tasty!"

I agree that cooked food can be tasty. But wait a minute, could you do me a favor today? Try cooking the best, most flavorful food you can without adding any **salt**.

If you're not the one cooking, ask your partner or even your favorite chef at your preferred restaurant to prepare something incredibly delicious, but with one catch: **no salt**. You might get some puzzled looks from your partner or the chef.

I would love you to share your experience with me and explain the taste of cooked food without salt. Imagine what taste you would get from cooked food without adding salt and/or spices. Salt in excess acts like a toxin with its strong taste. While our bodies need sodium and chloride in small amounts, we naturally obtain them from fruits and some vegetables. We rarely require additional salt in a raw lifestyle.

In a natural lifestyle with Raw Vegan (Raw Fruitarian) eating, you don't need salt and spices to enhance the taste of your plate. The natural ingredients are inherently flavorful and satisfying, requiring no additional flavors or salt.

Have you noticed the pleasant smell of cooked food? How does the smell of the delicious dinner your partner prepared welcome you when you come back home from work? That wonderful smell is often the beneficial nutrition escaping into the air, while the authentic taste of the raw ingredients is lost through heating. This often leaves us craving the remaining salty and spicy materials.

Chefs enhance the taste of heat-treated foods with various methods and ingredients such as salt, chili, spices, garlic, and onion. Anyone can discern the true nature of cooked food by eliminating these additives.

While heating does create strong aromas and new flavours through processes such as the Maillard reaction, this comes at a cost: heat-sensitive vitamins, antioxidants, and enzymes are lost in the process. Although cooking may increase the bioavailability of certain compounds like lycopene in tomatoes or beta-carotene in carrots, it simultaneously reduces vitamin C, B vitamins, and delicate enzymes that are essential for health. Minerals may be more stable, but even they can oxidise or leach out into cooking water.

You can try it tonight. Take **a fresh** and ripe fruit with its **authentic taste**, place it in a pot, cook it for a while, and taste the difference. I would love to hear about your experience.

On another note, have you noticed that many food items from the supermarket advise storing them in sealed containers away from heat and sunlight? Have you ever wondered why this is necessary? The answer lies in preventing oxidation, which can render them toxic and tasteless.

Also, why do we keep most food materials in a fridge? Why do we need a cooler environment to keep them fresh (not oxidised)?

It is ironic that we carefully keep our raw materials cool and fresh, only to expose them to high heat just before eating. If heating were truly beneficial, why would we need fridges at all? By that logic, we could store our food in a running oven.

Next time you're about to buy bread, think of it as 'wheat that's already been through the oven once.' Or when dining out, imagine telling the waiter you'd like their best 'heat-treated cuisine.' It makes you smile, but it also makes you wonder about the true origin of the taste!

What is Disease?

"All diseases begin in the gut."

Hippocrates, the father of medicine

D isease happens when our organs cannot perform their normal functions. Pain is often one of the key signs of a disease, although not the only one.

How we feel is one of the most crucial indicators. When we lose the normal function of our body and do not feel good, it shows that something is not right.

Many factors can contribute to feeling unwell, and among these, food intake is one of the most important. Let us discuss some of them, mainly believed to be a source of feeling unwell or sickness.

Microbes and Viruses

Modern medical science believes most illnesses happen because some viruses or microbes attack us. This can sometimes be true, but can we realistically eliminate these little creatures from our lives?

Often, when no clear microbial cause is found, the explanation shifts to genetics. This can also hold truth, but we should ask:

where do we get our genes from? From our parents, of course. And what were the habits of our parents when we were created? And their parents before them?

Notice how effortlessly we place responsibility on others' shoulders. For example, blaming traffic when arriving late at an important appointment. What about blaming our parents for our poor financial situation? And when it comes to our health, who is responsible for it: the government, our doctor, the medical industry, or these little creatures, viruses and microbes? Or do we acknowledge that our lifestyle and choices also play a central role?

How do medical experts view our lifestyle? Do they study everyone to see what they eat and drink every day to discover the actual source of their problems? I understand this is not their duty sometimes, but what about us? Isn't it our job to reflect on our habits and establish a healthier lifestyle by modifying or eliminating harmful ones?

You might have heard that consuming alcohol can have a significant influence on pregnancy, potentially causing genetic problems in an unborn child due to its toxicity. But what about heat-damaged foods? Have you ever considered their impact? What effects do food-borne toxins have on the fetus and its genes? Unfortunately, the health of our genes has been compromised over generations due to the unhealthy lifestyles of our ancestors. Can we take steps to reduce or even reverse these effects for the benefit of future generations?

Returning to our discussion, microbes and viruses always live around us. Even in a pristine kitchen, they inhabit the fridge, dishes, sinks, and cutlery. Our body is designed intelligently enough to protect itself from these little creatures with several layers of protection called the immune system

The immune system adapts, recognising new harmful microbes and viruses, ensuring human survival. The issue happens when we weaken our excellent defense mechanism through our behaviors, especially our eating habits. The immune system, alongside other organs involved in digestion, must work hard to eliminate nutrient-compromised foods from our bodies. At the same time, when we consistently eat the wrong foods, we fail to provide proper nutrition to our immune system, leaving it weaker over time.

Modern research shows that around 70 percent of the immune system is located in the gut. This means diet is not just important, it is the primary influence on immunity. A healthy gut environment, supported by natural raw foods, helps the immune system recognise, fight, and adapt to microbes effectively.

A lot of people only think about eliminating microbes and viruses but may never consider how they can strengthen their immune system by providing it with proper fuel. I'm not suggesting that you shouldn't wash your hands or maintain good hygiene practices. On the contrary, it's crucial that we make every effort to minimise the chances of harmful microbes or viruses entering our bodies. This reduces the load on the immune system and gives time for the organs involved in elimination to rest.

While we may minimise the intake of harmful microbes, we simultaneously place significant strain on our organs by feeding them improperly. This forces them to work tirelessly to eliminate the oxidised foods we consume most of the time.

When our immune system is compromised by consuming heat-damaged foods, we are at risk, and any viruses or microbes, even in small quantities, can grow fast in our bodies and create diseases.

Intoxicated Body

The materials we consume can also create problems directly within our bodies. Our level of health is closely influenced by what we introduce each day through food and drink.

During high-temperature cooking or heavy processing, several compounds can form, including aldehydes, acrylamide, polycyclic aromatic hydrocarbons (PAHs), heterocyclic amines (HCAs), advanced glycation end products (AGEs), trans fatty acids, nitrosamines, and even furan. These substances have been studied for their potential to contribute to oxidative stress and other imbalances in the body.

Some of the **oxidised compounds**, called *free radicals*, are created by heating raw materials. Cooking, especially with high heat, generates free radicals in large amounts, which become a major driver of oxidative stress, contributing to early aging and many diseases. It has been clear from several pieces of research (see References) that cancer and cardiovascular diseases (CVD) often occur due to free-radical damage, and these two diseases are major causes of human death.

Naturally, free radicals are created in our bodies by cell metabolism. The immune system also creates free radicals to destroy pathogens such as viruses and unwanted bacteria. The liver makes free radicals to be used for detoxification. However, in these cases, the body produces them in a controlled way and only as needed. In contrast, introducing fire to food, special at high temperature can create uncontrolled free radicals and sometimes in large quantities, often overwhelming our antioxidant reserves.

Free radicals or oxidant materials have one unpaired electron in their atom orbit and are unstable and highly reactive. They aggressively look to give or steal that one electron to become stable.

They usually have a short life; however, during this time they can significantly damage our bodies. Most of the time, they damage cell membranes or DNA by stealing their electrons.

On the flip side, antioxidants sacrifice themselves to give their electron to these free radicals to protect the cells. The human body produces some antioxidants, which are stable enough molecules to donate an electron to the free radicals and neutralise them.

Other antioxidants, such as Vitamin C, Vitamin E, and beta-carotene, are widely found in fresh fruits and vegetables and can help our bodies neutralise free radicals. Unfortunately, many of these antioxidants are damaged by heat and lose much of their effectiveness; sometimes even becoming **pro-oxidants** rather than protectors.

When a free radical steals an electron from a healthy cell, it can turn that cell into a free radical too, continuing the destructive chain reaction. This is one of the reasons people look in the mirror and feel upset at how quickly their skin ages; often trying to mask it with makeup products, a temporary fix we all know too well. But while skin and eyes reveal some damage, what about the *countless internal cells you cannot see?*

Returning to our discussion about toxins, by eating and drinking, we introduce some into our bodies every day, even when following a proper natural lifestyle. How does this happen? Firstly, small amounts of oxidants occur naturally in raw foods. These can form when fruits or vegetables are cut, peeled, or exposed to air and sunlight. However, raw foods come packed with powerful antioxidants such as Vitamin C, flavonoids, and polyphenols, which far outweigh and neutralise these minor oxidants. This natural balance supports health rather than harms it.

The real problem begins when food is subjected to prolonged heating, especially at high temperatures, which not only destroys many of those antioxidants but also generates quite large amounts of new free radicals.

In addition, toxins may also be present in raw materials due to chemical residues, fertilisers, pesticides, polluted air and water, soil contamination, and even from food containers. People who follow a Raw diet may also unknowingly consume toxins from these sources, including chlorine in drinking water and exhaust gases in the air. Finally, some toxins are also produced internally as waste byproducts of the body's own metabolism.

Naturally, our body has **mechanisms to handle** these toxins and eliminate them through the lymphatic and digestive systems. This detoxification capacity is limited by the capabilities of the organs involved in detoxification including the lymphatic system, liver, veins, and kidneys. When toxin levels exceed what our bodies can process, the digestive system may store them inside our bodies. Common storage locations for toxins include soft tissues like fat cells, breasts, under the skin, and glands such as the liver, pancreas, and thyroid. Joints can also serve as sites for toxin accumulation.

To understand it better, imagine we have a tank with 100 litres of water capacity. The tank has a valve with a maximum capacity of delivering 1 litre per hour of water. It means the tap can deliver 24 litres of water per 24 hours.

If we put 24 litres of water inside the tank and leave the tap fully open, then at the end of the day (after 24 hours), all water will be emptied, and no water will remain in the tank. If we put less than 24 litres of water inside the tank and leave the tap open, the tank will be emptied sooner than 24 hours.

If we put more than 24 litres, say 30 litres per day, inside the tank and leave the tap fully open after 24 hours, guess what happens? Yes, correct. We will have 6 litres remaining inside the tank. After ten days, 60 litres will accumulate. After 20 days, the tank overflows because it has only 100 litres capacity.

The same thing happens in our body. When our body cannot process and eliminate all the toxins, the surplus will be stored within. If we put in more than the storage capacity of our body, then we start vomiting or getting diarrhea, which is our body's defense mechanism to get rid of the extra toxins as quickly as possible. Or we lose our desire for food altogether, which is another mechanism our body uses to minimise the toxic intake.

Have you ever noticed a sudden wave of nausea without any obvious reason? If so, did you ever stop to ask yourself why you felt that way? Often, it is the body's natural warning signal, a way of saying, "I've had enough, please stop loading me with more unhealthy foods."

In the tank example mentioned earlier, another way to increase the amount of water intake is to increase the capacity of the tank. Similarly, our bodies can expand in size to accommodate increased toxin levels. Consider how regular consumption of junk food and soft drinks can lead to weight gain. One role of fat is to act as a reservoir for storing certain substances, and while not the only cause of obesity, it partly explains why our bodies pack on more fat when overloaded with toxins.

Have you ever noticed a lack of hunger after consuming fast food for an extended period? Some individuals may even experience symptoms such as nausea or vomiting. In such cases, they may seek medical help from their general practitioner (GP), who might prescribe medication to alleviate symptoms like vomiting or diarrhea by temporarily paralysing the nerves responsible. It's a bit like putting duct tape over a smoke alarm instead of putting out the fire.

You may have had the experience or seen someone fully intoxicated with alcohol, and their body is trying to get rid of the extra alcohol (toxic) by vomiting it out. Another mechanism the body employs to limit toxin intake is to induce feelings of sickness when there is little space left in tissues, glands, and joints. As mentioned earlier, have you ever noticed that food becomes unappealing when feeling unwell?

When sick, people are often urged to eat even if they have no hunger. I remember the struggles I faced as a child, forced to eat steak (considered powerful food) when I was unwell. Ironically, the "power food" intended to help battle sickness often made me feel worse. In reality, the best cure was to rest the body and abstain from eating until it had reset itself.

If you disregard the signals and persist in eating, your body will expand its capacity, often by creating fat cells and storing water between tissues. This is a primary reason why some people who consume excessive junk food tend to gain size through increased fat cell production and water retention.

The additional water stored between tissues serves two functions: expanding the body's capacity and diluting toxins to mitigate their effects. Now you can see why obesity is spreading so widely today, and sadly, even children are affected at an age when their bodies should be light, active, and free.

The storage of toxins creates problems for the glands and interrupts their functions. People get diabetes because the pancreas cannot work well due to the damage of beta cells producing insulin and can be easily damaged by free radicals, and extra fat prevents insulin from entering the cells and burning the sugar.

From natural hygiene perspective high cholesterol and cirrhosis happen when the liver gets injured by harmful substances and loses its proper function; fatty liver is another result. Arthritis can develop when waste products build up in the joints.

You may go to the doctor, and after a couple of tests, they give you medications to put the glands back to work. I understand that medications can sometimes help reduce symptoms and give the body time to heal itself. From time to time, they may assist certain organs in performing their functions more effectively. While I do appreciate the contributions of medical science and doctors in improving human life, it's important to recognise that the chemicals in pills and drugs can potentially harm other organs and cause side effects.

In many cases, medications mainly manage symptoms instead of addressing root causes. Sometimes they may delay the illness, but when it returns it often comes back stronger, requiring stronger prescriptions. This cycle can continue for years, almost like upgrading to the next "level" of medicine instead of breaking free from the game altogether.

A teenager may not realise the long-term effects of cooked and processed foods on their health. Their youthful bodies can often tolerate a certain amount of unhealthy inputs, leading only to occasional sickness. Children and young adults are typically more active than older humans, which can bolster their immune system, circulation, and digestion, helping them cope with some of the strain.

However, if you're young and believe you can handle all the cooked, processed and unhealthy foods you consume, consider observing older adults, especially your parents or grandparents, who may have followed a similar lifestyle. It is almost like peeking into a time machine: their health today may offer a glimpse of where your own choices could lead tomorrow.

Unfortunately, many people believe that illness, hospitalisation, surgery, **organ removal**, and medication are inevitable aspects of life. They perceive these health complications as normal occurrences.

One of my older, close family members showed me her bag of tablets she took every day. To my shock, she was consuming around 18 different pills daily! This didn't even include the extra sorbents and supplements she regularly took.

She had medications for high blood pressure, vertigo, high cholesterol, thyroid function, arthritis, and various other conditions. She mentioned that she began with just one or two tablets per day years ago and gradually escalated to taking more than 100 pills per week.

Was she cured? Not at all. Did the medications help her? Yes, but mostly by reducing symptoms rather than addressing the root causes.

The challenge with medications is that while they often target one problem, they can create side effects elsewhere. A common example is antibiotics. They are frequently prescribed to eliminate bacteria and viruses, which are believed to be the sources of illness. While antibiotics can be very effective at killing harmful pathogens, they also destroy many of the beneficial bacteria in our gut. And those friendly microbes aren't just passengers, they are essential for digestion, nutrient absorption, and overall health. It's a bit like hiring someone to fix a leaky tap, only to find out they've turned off the entire water supply in your house.

I remember a couple of years ago, after being fully Raw Vegan and following my natural lifestyle for years, I visited my dentist to get an implant. Unfortunately, I damaged some of my nice teeth when I was young with the wrong lifestyle, eating junk foods and drinking alcohol. After implanting, my professional dentist prescribed me some antibiotics to be taken.

It was just three pills, one each day for three days. I mentioned to her that I hadn't taken medicine for many years. I was deeply reluctant to take the medicine; however, she insisted and said it was like a minor surgery, and I must take the medicine; otherwise, there wouldn't be any guarantee that the implants would stay there if any infections occurred in the affected area. I had a tough time convincing myself to listen to her and, unfortunately, took the pills.

You can't imagine what happened. My body's reaction was extreme. I experienced severe constipation for about a week, something I had never encountered before in my life.

I felt terrible during that period and couldn't perform my daily tasks, leading me to take days off from work. It felt like my gut was staging a rebellion, and trust me, it won.

It was then that I realised what a big mistake I had made. With proper fasting and increased physical exercise over the course of a couple of weeks, I was finally able to overcome the issue. It was a painful experience, one that I'll never forget and certainly never repeat. I was fortunate the medication was only for a short period. But it left me wondering: what happens to people who take pills not for three days, but for years, even decades, hoping to reclaim their health?

Now, let me ask you a simple question: while our body's ability to eliminate harmful substances is limited, why do we keep adding even more by subjecting food to prolonged high heat? Why add free radicals, aldehydes, and acrylamides on top of it all; especially when combined with processed and junk foods?

Please remember, no one else can heal your body; it heals itself. Especially when you are sick, the best support you can give is time, rest, and nourishing fuel, while avoiding the unnecessary things that weigh it down.

Chronic Diseases

Many diseases develop gradually and return frequently enough that they eventually become chronic. Too often, we try to manage them only by reducing the symptoms. But because the underlying causes remain; especially heavily processed or heat-damaged foods that place extra strain on the body; the problems keep coming back and sometimes grow stronger.[1]

Many health conditions are labeled as incurable by the medical industry. Alzheimer's[2], CVD[3], arthritis, asthma and diabetes are some examples.

Cancer provides another case where cells can spread and grow due to long-term damage and the build-up of harmful substances in our bodies. When poor diet and lifestyle weaken the immune system, it struggles to regulate and eliminate abnormal cells as effectively as it should.

Proper nutrition, including essential nutrients like selenium and Vitamin D, is crucial for supporting the immune system in producing protective cells.

---

[1] Can sometimes be genetic disorders.

[2] Alzheimer's disease is a progressive neurological disorder that primarily affects memory, thinking, and behavior. (see Glossary)

[3] Cardiovascular diseases – Related to the heart and blood vessels. (see Glossary)

According to science, cancer cells can potentially develop in anyone's body due to various factors such as free radicals, radiation, genetic predisposition, and ultraviolet (UV) exposure. These can all trigger changes at the cellular level.

However, our immune system has the remarkable capability to detect and remove these abnormal cells. The problem is that this defense mechanism becomes overworked and less effective when constantly exposed to poor nutrition and modern eating habits. For people following the Typical Western Diet (T.W.D.), filled with processed foods and meals cooked at high temperatures, the immune system is under ongoing strain without much chance of recovering.

When this protective system becomes exhausted, it grows weaker and less prepared to deal with the microbes and viruses constantly present around us. Overworked by coping with poor diet and damaged foods, the immune system struggles to maintain its defences, allowing diseases, including abnormal cell growth such as cancer to develop and spread more easily.

High levels of harmful buildup in different organs can cause specific problems:

- In the pancreas: this can impair its ability to produce enough beta cells, which are essential for helping insulin move glucose into the body's cells. Over time, this can lead to diabetes.
- In the liver: accumulation may contribute to fatty liver, cirrhosis, and poor liver function, often accompanied by elevated cholesterol levels.
- In the joints: deposits and inflammation can contribute to arthritis or rheumatoid arthritis (RA).
- In the veins and capillaries: this can interfere with blood flow, contributing to migraines and cardiovascular disease.

Asthma, multiple sclerosis (MS), and Parkinson's are other conditions that may be influenced by long-term consumption of poor-quality or heavily processed foods.

- **Asthma:** When the lungs are exposed to repeated irritation from poor-quality foods, preservatives, and chemical additives, their capacity to function can become compromised. For example, sulphur compounds, widely used in the food and special wine industry, can inflame or irritate lung tissue. Many people drink wine regularly, believing that wine; especially red wine is healthy. Over time, this repeated exposure can set the stage for asthma or make existing breathing difficulties worse, often leading to reliance on steroid sprays.

- **Multiple sclerosis (MS):** Although MS is often described as an autoimmune disease, diet and lifestyle appear to play important roles in how it progresses. When the body is constantly exposed to oxidised fats, processed sugars, and chemicals, the immune system may misfire and begin attacking its own tissues. The nervous system, which is especially delicate, can suffer from inflammation and poor cellular repair when it is deprived of the nutrients it needs.

- **Parkinson's disease:** Emerging research suggests that oxidative stress, mitochondrial damage, and chronic inflammation may contribute to Parkinson's. Diets high in processed and heat-damaged foods can increase oxidative stress and deprive the nervous system of protective antioxidants. Over time, this can accelerate nerve cell injury, which is a hallmark of Parkinson's.

While genetics, environment, and other factors can play a role in these conditions, diet and lifestyle choices remain a powerful lever for reducing risk and supporting better outcomes. It is not about claiming food alone is the cause but recognising that what we eat can either fuel the fire of disease or help put it out.

The cells we build today with the foods we eat will either support health and clarity or contribute to disease and decline tomorrow. When a new cell is created, it is crucial to consider the quality of the nutrients it receives. If the new cell is nourished with ultra-processed or heat-damaged foods, it may develop into a weakened or compromised cell. Conversely, if it receives genuine and nutritious food, it will become a healthy cell. Which would you prefer? A robust, healthy cell or a struggling one? The choice is yours.

Weakened or poorly nourished cells cannot function properly and may contribute to chronic conditions, including cancer and autoimmune issues such as MS. Some health problems also arise from our body's reaction to substances it cannot process efficiently, leading to strain or injury in internal organs. Our body communicates with us through pain, discomfort, or digestive upset. If these early signals are overlooked, the underlying issues may progress, sometimes showing up later as more persistent problems such as chronic headaches or even migraines. Persisting with unhealthy eating habits over time increases the risk of serious disease.

When we visit doctors, they may prescribe medications to manage symptoms and stabilise conditions. While these can be life-saving in many situations, some medicines also come with side effects. Certain pain medications, for example, dampen nerve signals so discomfort feels reduced, but this does not resolve the underlying cause. Fortunately, many healthcare professionals today are also looking deeper, recommending lifestyle changes and holistic approaches to address root causes.

Our body is remarkably adaptive and resilient, often accommodating less-than-ideal diets. Unlike putting diesel into a petrol car, which causes immediate failure, our bodies can process a wide variety of "fuels," though sometimes at a cost. The extent of that cost varies from person to person, depending on genetics, environment, and lifestyle.

Enzymes

Enzymes are typically proteins and are essential for food digestion. They act as catalysts, breaking food down into smaller molecules and particles for our body's absorption and use by our cells.

Raw foods naturally contain enzymes that support digestion and absorption. However, when prolonged high heat is applied to these foods, many of their natural enzymes are damaged or destroyed.

It's true that our body can produce the enzymes it needs. But this requires extra effort from our organs, placing more demand on them and using additional energy. Why make your organs work overtime when raw foods can bring their own "helpers" to the job? It's a bit like having kitchen staff already chopping and prepping; why send them home and do all the hard work yourself?

Research (see References) suggests that our body's enzyme activity can decline with age. This is one reason older adults often experience digestive challenges and reduced stomach function. When digestion becomes less efficient, the body struggles to extract vitamins and minerals from food. Over time, deficiencies in key nutrients may contribute to a wide range of health problems.

Many people also report feelings of nervousness, frustration, or anxiety without fully understanding the underlying cause. In some cases, poor nutrient absorption from impaired digestion may play a role in these feelings, though it is not the only factor.

Have you heard about the interconnection between body and mind, and how the gut signals discomfort to the brain?

When your digestive system is not working well, key nutrients such as **magnesium**, **B vitamins**, and **potassium** may not be absorbed efficiently. These are all critical for healthy nerve function. A shortage of them can sometimes contribute to feelings of anxiety, irritability, or low mood.

As a result, people may seek medical advice and begin taking antidepressant tablets. While these can provide temporary relief, they may also bring side effects and, in some cases, dependency. Others approach the issue as purely psychological and consult a psychologist. They may then be prescribed tranquilizers to calm the nerves and reduce signals of anxiety.

Please remember an earlier point: disease is often the body's way of signalling that something in our behaviour is off balance. Many medicines act more like "mute buttons," suppressing those signals rather than addressing the root cause.

Several chronic conditions are strongly tied to poor gut function. Insufficient absorption of vitamins and minerals can lead to fatigue, impaired vision, arthritis, cardiovascular issues, high blood pressure, diabetes, and elevated cholesterol. While medicines may sometimes help the digestive system in the short term, long-term reliance can reduce its natural function.

To wrap up this chapter, losing enzymes through heat treatment of foods can gradually wear down the digestive system, leading to nutrient deficiencies and illness. Disease is not random; it begins as your body whispering for change. Ignore it, and over time, those whispers become shouts; especially about what you put on your plate.

Nothing can heal a disease except the body itself. With proper nourishment, the body has the tools to repair and function at its best.

Dr Robert Morse, in his book "The Detox Miracle Sourcebook", says: We have two choices to make when we develop a condition or disease:

- **Treatment**

   or

- **Detoxification**

You have the freedom to choose. Opting for treatment may mean a lifelong commitment, sometimes with uncertain permanence.

In my view, treatment is often necessary, and in many cases it should work hand in hand with detoxification, at least for **a period of time**.

Capture 5

Medical Industry

In many cases, the medical industry has done remarkable work. Doctors, nurses, pharmacists, and medicine factories have contributed greatly to human health, especially in identifying the causes of new diseases, treating accident victims, performing necessary surgeries, and managing pregnancy complications. They have also carried out extensive research on human nutrition and created supplements that have proven useful in many situations.

Medical science has advanced enormously over the past centuries, often with significant human effort and sacrifice. Countless hours of research, product development, examinations, and tests have brought real progress. However, much of this progress has focused on treatments and cures rather than on understanding and preventing the root causes of disease. Sometimes, the solutions offered provide only temporary relief, mainly by removing or suppressing symptoms.

We are often presented with chemical tablets, capsules, or liquid medicines for pain relief. Surgeries, chemotherapy, and radiotherapy can certainly remove diseased or unhealthy cells. These interventions can be lifesaving and sometimes give the body the space it needs to begin its own healing process. Yet, the results are not always consistent or permanent.

Take the example of a tumour. Surgery can remove it, but if the underlying cause is not identified and corrected, another tumour may form, sometimes larger than the first. When we only treat the signs without addressing the root problem, the cycle continues.

It is similar with conditions like high blood pressure. Medication can lower the numbers on a test result, but if diet, stress, or lifestyle remains unchanged, the underlying issue is still there. The pills manage the numbers, but they do not fix the cause.

It is much like having a leaky roof. You can put a bucket underneath to catch the water, and for a while it looks like the problem is solved. But as the leak worsens, you keep reaching for a bigger bucket. The real solution, of course, is not a bigger bucket, it is *fixing the roof*.

None of the patients want to progress from stage 1 to stage 4 of cancer, but unfortunately, it often occurs when lifestyle changes are not made alongside medical treatment. Generally, medications may only temporarily alleviate symptoms without addressing the underlying causes. And since many of these causes are lifestyle-related, they cannot simply be erased with medication alone. How can we expect to fully resolve a root problem if we only manage the surface symptoms?

Another example, when experiencing a headache, one might purchase a painkiller from a pharmacist or supermarket. The pill may bring quick relief by blocking or dulling the nerve signals to the brain. But the relief is short-lived, and the cycle of pain often continues. The medicine handles the signal, but not always the message. It is essential to also investigate and address the root cause of the pain. Unfortunately, this step is often overlooked.

I have observed that much less emphasis is placed on prevention and on understanding the true sources of disease than on finding treatments. Some argue that the reason is commercial, with far more funds allocated to cures than to prevention.

You may agree that prevention is far better than cure because it can stop an issue before it develops. When treatment is needed, it should ideally be directed at the root of the problem, not only at its signs and signals.

That said, I fully acknowledge that medications are sometimes necessary. They can be **life-saving** in the short term, such as during surgery after an accident or when complications arise in pregnancy. In these cases, modern medicine shines, and its role is invaluable.

Medicines can sometimes have side effects and harm other organs. Years ago, when I was younger, I was prescribed diclofenac infusions to relieve unbearable pain. It was a common drug back then, and I was grateful for its effectiveness. A couple of years later, when I revisited my doctor for the same issue and asked for diclofenac, it was no longer available. With a smile, he informed me that it had been banned in many places due to its potential for serious kidney and cardiovascular damage.

How often have you heard of a medicine being banned or restricted because of long-term side effects? Imagine if we could address health issues at their source and prevent them in the first place. In such cases, relying less on medications might be preferable, considering the risks that sometimes come with them.

What if the medical industry worked just as hard on uncovering the root causes of disease, rather than focusing mainly on creating stronger medicines by mixing and combining chemicals?

I recall a TV ad years ago that promoted a tablet for a "better digestive system." The ad showed people rushing through their lunch, especially fast foods, and suffering stomach pain. The solution? Take the tablet before eating so you could keep eating fast without pain. Have you ever wondered why anyone would take a pill to eat faster instead of simply slowing down? It's a little ironic, isn't it? Swallowing chemicals just to keep swallowing food more quickly!

As I've said before, pain is not the enemy. Pain is a signal, part of your body's own language telling you that something is wrong. By changing your lifestyle, behaviour, and especially your eating habits, you can reduce or even eliminate many of these signals. You don't need to **paralyse** your body's alarm system with tablets when sometimes the answer is as simple as chewing more slowly and letting your stomach keep its dignity.

Capture 6

Length or Width

Sometimes, when I shared the story of having a proper natural lifestyle to live a real healthy life, some people's responses were:

"I don't care; I don't want to change my lifestyle and special my diet and love cooked food. I eat and drink whatever I like and can get from supermarket shelves. I am happy to live five years less if it happens with unhealthy food and soft drinks!" or

"I want to enjoy my life even if it is the shortest!"

Which one is more significant: the length or width of life? You could live to 120 years or more, but if much of that time is spent sick, running from one hospital to another, and not enjoying life, especially after the age of 60 or 70, then what is the value? Quality matters just as much as quantity.

Imagine you have a fleet of old cars, all with a bunch of issues. One has a faulty brake, and another has a non-functioning steering wheel. You are spending all your energy and money trying to fix them one after the other, but none of them get fixed well enough to be reliable for a pleasant journey or to tow your caravan to a camp.

Now imagine someone offers to replace them with a brand-new, reliable car with modern functions and no issues. Would you hesitate? It is the same for our bodies. Which one is better for our life journey, a healthy, strong and reliable body that can be taken anywhere without fear of getting sick often, which can ruin our trip? Or a bunch of unhealthy organs that require various medications and occasional hospital visits?

Our life is not guaranteed for tomorrow; but, if you are allowed to live for only one day, would you prefer to live it fully with a robust body with all its healthy organs? Or being sick and bed-bound?

If you are young, you may feel energised because your body has not yet been overloaded with unhealthy habits, and you might think you are doing fine despite a few health issues. But pause and look ahead. What does life look like at your middle age or after 60? If you think you will escape decline, look at your parents and grandparents. Their health may be your preview if you continue the same lifestyle.

I believe we need to enjoy every second of our lives, and our healthy bodies have the most critical role in our entire journey. It's all about our feelings, and feelings always happen inside. When we are nice to our bodies, give them the proper fuel, and take care of them, we feel great and have a wonderful life. It doesn't matter how long we are going to live.

You may have noticed how you feel inside when your digestive system works appropriately. In contrast, remember when you ran into constipation and had difficulty eliminating the waste. Which one gives you a better feeling? Or how does it feel to be in your standard body shape compared to when you were overweight and carrying extra fats all the time?

In addition, with your natural lifestyle, it looks like you are running on an energy booster. As we have already discussed, high energy levels are created by consuming live and real food rather than processed or heavily oxidised ones. This vitality gives you momentum to face life's challenges more easily.

Since I started this natural living journey, I have felt at least 15 years younger due to my excellent energy levels.

This transformation is not unique to me; thousands of people following the same lifestyle have experienced similar benefits, with some reducing their biological age even more than I have. The difference depends on how much damage the body has carried and how quickly it can cleanse.

Have you noticed that you have a wonderful feeling when your energy is high? Many people feel great when they go to nature and boost their energy. Others boost their energy with alcohol or drugs and feel good temporarily. Even though alcohol artificially stimulates our energy for a short period, and when the effect wears off, the crash follows(sometimes with a headache), people still love drinking because it makes them feel better in the moment.

What if you could feel amazing all the time just by consuming the food intended for you by nature, without relying on drinking alcohol? And for some people with smoking or even drugs?

Many individuals with T.W.D. (Typical Western Diet) think they are healthy and feel OK. If you are one of them, I suggest considering your feelings when you wake up in the morning. Do you need an alarm to wake up? If so, consider whether that is natural. Do you know of any other creature in nature that uses an alarm clock? Also, how is your sleep? Do you need a tranquiliser to go to sleep? Or coffee to keep you awake in the mornings?

These questions are critical for assessing your true health and determining how your **organs are performing**.

If you want to gauge your health, consider observing yourself first thing in the morning when you wake up, looking at your face in the mirror, makeup-free. How does your face appear? Do you notice puffiness, especially under your eyes? Skin and eyes are the most sensitive organs showing internal conditions; it is easy to determine whether you are in optimal health by examining them when you wake up.

With a proper natural lifestyle and by consuming foods designed by nature, you may find that you wake up without needing an alarm, and your skin appears radiant in the morning. Your senses are heightened, and you may not feel the need for stimulants to reawaken and feel energised.

When you start your natural way of living by incorporating more raw food daily, your senses, especially taste and smell, sharpen and you rediscover the true flavours of food. Experience the true essence of raw ingredients for enhanced happiness.

The above explanation outlines how the quality of your life can improve by a natural lifestyle, now let's discuss quantity.

I believe that with a proper lifestyle and diet, you can achieve a longer lifespan. While no research exists on life expectancy for humans following a Raw lifestyle, we can look to nature for some insights. Many animals, with the right diet, live longer than humans.

For instance, chimpanzees, whose DNA is closest to that of humans, live approximately 50-60 years while reaching maturity at 6 or 7 years old. This means they live roughly ten times their maturity age. By comparison, if a human reaches maturity at 14-15 years old, they should theoretically live about 130-150 years. I mean active life, not living with mechanical aids or being bedridden in a hospital.

Horses have a lifespan of 25 years and reach maturity at 18 months. This suggests that humans should live around 240-250 years.

Having a short life, as humans have these days, did not happen overnight. For years and generations, our wrong food intake and inappropriate lifestyle have compromised our genes and weakened our body cells, and we are what we are now. From my point of view, living much longer than life expectancy will take time for the whole human race, but as an individual, we can live longer with the proper fuel designed for us compared to eating the wrong one.

Picture a longer, fulfilling life with a balanced lifestyle and harmony with nature. Embrace every moment with energy and optimism, knowing that better days lie ahead.

I hope I could address the concerns of the ones thinking of the wrong lifestyle and fuel. When someone says they are enjoying their unhealthy lifestyle, I wonder; are they really enjoying it, or are they just trading tomorrow's health for today's habits?!

Capture 7

Detoxification

You may have noticed that athletes are generally healthier than others. Do you know why? Some people believe it's because physical activity improves mental health, which in turn supports the body. Others suggest that athletes simply have better metabolism. Let's look a little deeper.

Our body has two primary distribution and collection systems: the bloodstream and the lymphatic. The bloodstream distributes nutrients and oxygen to the cells, while the lymphatic system collects excess fluid, waste products, and toxins from the tissues. The lymph then transports these waste products to lymph nodes, where they are filtered out, and eventually returns the filtered lymph back into the bloodstream or directs it to other organs, such as the digestive tract, for elimination of the waste.

To understand the two systems, consider the bloodstream as a building's freshwater supply network and the lymphatic system as its sewerage. Much like in a building, the bloodstream is circulated by a pump (the heart) which pushes blood through veins and capillaries, similar to how water is distributed through the piping in a structure.

In contrast, the lymphatic system acts like a building's sewerage, collecting waste, toxins, and excess fluids from tissues and organs and directing them to lymph nodes for filtration and disposal. Like sewage, the lymphatic system relies on gravity for proper functioning, while also benefiting from body movement. The more you move during the day, the better your lymphatic system works.

Movement helps to stimulate **lymph flow** and prevent fluid buildup, promoting overall lymphatic health. That is one reason health experts often recommend at least 30 minutes of daily activity; it is not just about burning calories but keeping your body's drainage system flowing. It is crucial for our health to be active.

If someone, because of disability, cannot move, then they need a regular massage to help their lymph system work. A disease called 'Bedsore' happens in patients who cannot move and must stay in bed for an extended period. These sores develop when prolonged pressure reduces blood and lymph circulation, leading to tissue damage. There are types of pressure-changing mattresses that are utilised under the patient, which work like a constant massage to prevent bedsores in non-moving patients, especially in the ICUs[1] in hospitals.

You might have experienced staying in bed longer than usual and noticed how your mood suffers when you wake up late. People often feel sluggish when they oversleep, especially if it becomes a habit over several days. This is because toxins can accumulate in the body with minimal body movement, affecting the functionality of the lymphatic system. It's your body's way of saying, "Nice nap, but I could use a little walk now!

Taking a cold shower can stimulate circulation and help support the detox process, or engaging in quick exercise can restore balance to the body. Some individuals even turn to coffee or alcohol as stimulants, but in reality these substances act as mild toxins, forcing the lymphatic system to work harder to flush them out alongside other waste products.

---

[1] Intensive Care Units in Hospitals which are for patients with critical conditions.

Detoxification is a continuous, natural process in our body. We constantly eliminate waste and byproducts through the digestive system, breathing, and sweating.

The digestive system has natural processes to clear residual food between meals. After food is digested in the stomach and pushed towards the small intestine, muscular contractions called peristalsis move the food along the digestive tract. During fasting periods (between meals), the migrating motor complex (MMC) helps sweep away any remaining food and debris in the stomach and intestines. This natural "housekeeping wave" is crucial, and frequent snacking disrupts it. Think of it like vacuuming a room; if you keep dropping crumbs, the job never gets done.

Our body has a limited capacity for detoxification, which depends on our body mass and the organs involved, including the lymph system, stomach, intestines and glands such as the liver and pancreas. As explained before, regular exercise dramatically influences our body's detoxification capacity.

However, this ability tends to decline with age as organs become less efficient. Here's the good news: when we minimise the intake of harmful substances, the body quickly shifts into a more powerful cleansing mode. This is what many people call a "detox." In simple terms, when you stop overloading the system, your body finally has the breathing space to catch up and repair itself.

Are you one of those who get headaches when you feel hungry? If so, have you questioned why it happens? You may think hunger is equal to headache, that is not always the case. When we pause food intake, which is what happens when we feel hungry and do not eat, the body often begins detoxifying. As stored byproducts are released into the bloodstream and lymph system, we can temporarily feel unwell, sometimes even developing headaches.

The (heavy) detox process begins from the first day we choose a proper natural lifestyle and may continue for sometimes, depending on the amount of waste materials stored in our bodies.

The initial 14 days were quite challenging for me, but I was prepared for this phase through research and conversations with others who had similar experiences. I drank a large amount of filtered water, took more rest than usual, and did frequent light exercises to help detoxification and cope with the changes.

Although I experienced several symptoms similar to those of the flu, the process was ultimately rewarding because I could sense my body working to eliminate stored toxins. At the same time, the healing began, and my overall mood started to improve.

I felt a lot lighter, something I missed from early childhood. Two weeks later, the initial symptoms were gone, but the detox continued for several months. People experience detoxification differently; however, most symptoms and durations are remarkably similar, even if the details vary from person to person.

For me, the major symptoms of detoxification disappeared within 8 weeks, and I could feel significant improvement in my overall **well-being**. That being said, I've had a couple of interesting experiences since then that I would like to share with you.

- After being fully Raw Vegan for about 18 months, I went into unexpected constipation, which was strange. I couldn't find a proper reason for it as I changed nothing in my diet or lifestyle. Then I noticed the signs of detox, and it continued for about ten days. When my body returned to its normal operation, I noticed many of the pains I was experiencing in my joints were all gone. I felt much more flexible, and I could do more activities with minimum pain in my knees, ankles, wrists, and elbows.

- Two years later, one morning I noticed a mark on my right eyelid when I looked at my face in the mirror. In the following day it developed and became a swelling. Initially, I was worried as it didn't look nice. Over two weeks, it grew larger, almost like a welt. I considered visiting my doctor, but since it caused no pain and I trusted the process, I waited to see what would happen.

  One morning, when I woke up and looked in the mirror, it had opened up, and fluid resembling white paste started flowing from it. This discharge continued for about two days before stopping, and the swelling disappeared. A couple of days later, it had fully healed, and my eyelid returned to its normal shape. I could not believe where my body had stored the toxins. In my right eyelid!

- Another interesting experience was when I celebrated my fourth year of being fully Raw. One morning, I noticed a lot of pain in my eyes. I ignored it for a couple of days, and gradually, the pain became intense. I decided to go for an eye test. The professional optometrist did several tests and said I have mild nearsightedness, and he recommended wearing spectacles for watching TV and reading. Before visiting him, I already knew about my nearsightedness since my teenage years.

  At some stage, when I was at university, I wore glasses for a couple of months; but my eyesight didn't change, and as it was mild, I discontinued the glasses. This time, I decided to use the spectacles to see if my severe eye pain was related to my nearsightedness. I wore the glasses for about a month, and the pain persisted. Then I noticed the colour of my eyes slightly shifted from dark brown to a brighter brown.

This was a remarkable change. My eyes looked younger, and I began researching online. I discovered that several Raw Vegans had reported similar changes. One of them is Kristina Carrillo-Bucaram, a writer, speaker, and Raw Vegan activist. Kristina uploaded a video on YouTube called *How My Eyes Changed Color Eating Fully Raw*, which I recommend watching.

It took me about eight weeks until my eye pain gradually disappeared, and the glasses didn't create any difference. I was amazed at how my organs were affected by years of unhealthy living and the detox process continued even after four years of being a fully Raw!

The eyes are one of our essential organs. Different parts of our eyes are connected to our internal organs, especially our intestines, and they are heavily affected by unhealthy buildup. It is one of the first organs to get affected by food or drink intake, and there are several signs and sicknesses our eyes show us we are affected. Notice how people's eyes indicate sickness, alcohol consumption, and drug use. Police officers are well aware of it!

From my understanding, the eyes are almost the last part of our body, which gradually detoxifies itself and many times changes its colours to a brighter version or even a different colour, which should be our original colour without the food we have introduced since birth.

Looking closely at a person's eyes can give hints about their overall health. Clear, bright eyes are often associated with vitality and youthfulness, while dullness, redness, or puffiness may suggest imbalance or strain. Although strong evidence for diet and detoxification permanently changing eye colour is limited, it is clear that proper nutrition, hydration, and a healthy lifestyle support eye health and can help maintain brightness and clarity.

Unfortunately, many people notice changes in their eyes, especially after middle age, which can be linked to years of lifestyle and diet choices. The next time you look in the mirror, don't just see your eyes; see them as a window into your true **state of health**.

Outcomes

So far, we have discussed the scientific reasons behind following our natural lifestyle and implementing a Raw diet. Now, I want to share the outcomes that can follow this choice. Let's explore them one by one.

Ultimate Health

The first and most important result of going Raw is what I call **Ultimate Health**. This means you may be free from many diseases and health complications and often won't need regular medication. Of course, outcomes depend on your existing health conditions, your genes, the degree of past damage to your body and critical organs from using the wrong fuel, and your daily habits.

People who adopt a natural diet with the right knowledge and guidance from professionals (especially if their health practitioner also values a natural lifestyle) often report remarkable changes. Some don't even get headaches and rarely need painkillers. You may only need to visit your GP or hospital for routine checkups, general consultations, or emergencies.

As soon as you stop damaging, the healing process begins. Depending on how quickly your body restores balance, your organs move closer to optimum health. Many people notice their stomach feels lighter, digestion improves, and they no longer rely on artificial stimulants like coffee or alcohol just to feel "normal." By embracing a natural lifestyle, you can experience lasting well-being while supporting your body, rather than harming it.

Your body can regain flexibility, often making you feel at least ten years younger than your actual age. Both body and mind benefit: when your digestive system is calm and efficient, your intestines can absorb nutrients more effectively, including essential ones like zinc. **Zinc** in particular plays a role in nervous system function and relaxation.

Another important outcome is *hormonal balance*. Most of us are familiar with how stress triggers the release of hormones like adrenaline and cortisol, which can disrupt health. But we often overlook the stress inside the body itself. Digestive stress can be constant, unlike external stress, which may only appear occasionally.

Many people live with low-level anxiety without understanding its source. They may turn to pills to feel calm. These can bring temporary relief, but as I mentioned earlier, chemicals can also add new burdens to the body over time. By contrast, a well-functioning digestive system reduces internal stress and helps maintain a steady sense of well-being. With a relaxed body, the likelihood of experiencing anxiety is greatly reduced, sometimes even eliminated altogether.

It's important to note that hormone secretion, such as adrenaline, in response to panic and stressful situations is a crucial part of our body's defense mechanism.

When faced with such situations, our body prepares for action by increasing blood flow to the muscles and accelerating the heartbeat, enabling us to either confront the threat or flee from it. The condition of our brain and our reactions are heavily influenced by these hormones.

Latest research (see References) suggests that we have significant number of neurons in our gut, which is why some scientists call it our "second brain." Serotonin, our 'feel-good' hormone, and dopamine, known as the 'bliss hormone,' are secreted in our digestive system in large quantities. The gut-brain axis, a complex communication network between the gastrointestinal tract and the central nervous system, plays a significant role in maintaining overall health and well-being.

Now think about these questions: How can a stressed or compromised gut consistently generate the right amounts of these hormones and truly make us feel good? Have you noticed your feeling when running into constipation? And how did you feel when the digestive tract works optimally?

An unhealthy lifestyle places strain on internal organs, preventing deep relaxation and often prompting people to turn to stimulants or sedatives such as **alcohol, coffee, and tranquillisers**. These may provide temporary relief by numbing nerves or blunting stress signals, but they further irritate the digestive system and make the long-term problem worse.

Another significant issue with a stressed digestive system is its impaired ability to absorb nutrients optimally. Key nutrients such as B group vitamins, zinc, and magnesium are vital for maintaining both a healthy body and a resilient nervous system. When absorption is compromised, the nervous system often weakens, and this can contribute to mental health issues including anxiety and depression.

You may now see more clearly how our body and mind are deeply interconnected, and why our food choices are crucial for our happiness. Our thoughts (the intake of the mind) can affect physical health, while poor food intake stresses the body and can fuel mental distress.

I've been asked: "If everyone lived a truly healthy life and stopped getting sick, what would happen to our economy? What about the medical industry, hospitals, doctors, and nurses? How would they earn their income? And what about the food industry, restaurants, cafes, and bars?"

Firstly, a healthier population could lead to increased productivity and reduced absenteeism in the workforce, which would have positive effects on the economy as a whole. Healthy individuals may also have more disposable income to spend on other goods and services, stimulating different sectors rather than just healthcare.

Furthermore, I don't believe any wise person would wish illness upon others. Doctors and nurses perform exceptional work, often sacrificing their own well-being to save lives. Most would be delighted to see fewer patients suffering, because their real mission is health, not sickness.

There is still much to be done by doctors, nurses, and hospitals: emergencies, accidents, pregnancy complications, regular check-ups, physical and mental consultations, and the list goes on. I always consult with our excellent family doctor and appreciate the valuable information he shares with me.

Many of my friends are medical doctors, and I have learned a great deal from them; their knowledge has been immensely beneficial in helping me find the right path to *Ultimate Health*.

At the same time, there is still relatively little research on the long-term benefits of natural lifestyles and optimal nutrition. How foods are transformed in our bodies and how different nutrients interact should be one of the great frontiers of science. Much more effort is needed to comprehend human natural needs, and this is a task perfectly suited to the **medical industry, scientists, and doctors.**

The food industry must also adapt to healthier lifestyles, including restaurants and cafes. They could create excellent natural meals for everyone and brand themselves as authentic restaurants, not just another fast-food stop.

Years ago, explaining what a vegetarian diet was would have been challenging. Yet today, vegetarian restaurants are common, reflecting the growing popularity of this lifestyle. A significant portion of the world's population now follows a vegetarian diet, and almost everyone has at least heard of it.

There is also a growing awareness of the vegan diet. Vegans follow stricter guidelines compared to vegetarians, avoiding all animal products. Several studies (see References) highlight the potential harm that excessive animal product consumption can cause. Many individuals report significant health benefits when adopting a vegan lifestyle.

It is estimated that there are more than 80 million vegans worldwide. There is potential for many of them to transition to a Raw Vegan diet once they realise how much nutrition is lost when food is oxidised and altered by heat.

Several restaurants are now offering Raw Vegan options alongside their cooked plates. Meeting people who are aware of Raw Veganism is promising, even if they are still relatively few. The good news is that Raw Vegan (Raw Fruitarian) and natural lifestyle followers are growing rapidly around the globe, and I am convinced this will be the future of our planet.

The transformation of industries to adapt to society's new condition is inevitable. There will always be important work for doctors, scientists, restaurants, and the food industry, only the focus will shift from sickness to wellness. And really, wouldn't that be a healthier business model for all?

Imagine a world where hospitals were known more for health education than for waiting rooms full of sick people. A world where restaurants proudly served fresh, vibrant meals that healed rather than harmed. Doesn't that sound like a future worth moving toward?

Healing

"Let food be thy medicine and medicine be thy food"

Hippocrates; the father of medicine

My understanding is that the vast majority of our diseases, perhaps 99%, come from what we eat, drink, breathe, or how we live our daily habits. These days, humans seem to eat almost everything! Walk into a supermarket and you'll be surprised at what is sold there as "food."

Many of the products on the shelves not only lack real benefits, but are also potentially harmful to our bodies once you look at their ingredients. For example, consider many soft drinks marketed as everyday beverages. If you check their labels, you'll see they are essentially sweetened water loaded with refined sugar, preservatives, artificial flavours, and colouring agents.

Some people even use them as household cleaning products! I've watched videos where these "soft drinks" are poured onto toilets or bathroom tiles as if they were powerful cleaners.

To understand how harsh they can be, try feeding one of your home plants with a soft drink and see how quickly it struggles.

Unlike plants, we are fortunate to have advanced physical bodies with digestive systems capable of handling these kinds of substances; at least for a while. But just because our bodies can process them doesn't mean they should. Constantly giving our digestive and immune systems extra work without proper rest weakens their ability to renew and protect us, eventually leading to illness.

Have you noticed that when you're sick, you lose your appetite and don't feel like eating or drinking? It's remarkable, isn't it? That's your body sending a signal: "Please stop feeding me, let me rest." This pause gives the immune system time to fight off the problem and restore balance. Yet, some health practitioners still encourage patients to eat so-called "power foods" to recover faster, which may actually place more strain on the body.

I remember as a young kid, I often fell ill. When my parents took me to our family doctor, he frequently suggested giving me steak as a "superfood" to regain strength. My kind mother would try to feed me, insisting it was good for me, but I had no appetite at all; it was painful and unpleasant. I hope you've never had the same experience, but if you have, you probably know how uncomfortable it felt.

Even in hospitals today, patients are still served items like soft drinks, muffins, and jellies. This shows how far we still have to go in recognising the importance of proper nutrition during recovery.

The healing process begins the moment we stop feeding the body harmful substances. Our intelligent bodies are always working to restore balance and return to their natural healthy state.

It is important to note that our bodies have a natural ability to heal themselves; external factors can only support this process. We need to give it time and proper nutrition, and sometimes nothing other than water, and let it heal itself. The problem is that many people neglect their physical well-being by not giving their bodies proper nutrition and constantly exposing themselves to harmful substances.

When we cease causing damage, the process reverses, and healing begins. This is why many people experience rapid recovery through a natural and proper lifestyle. Quite a large number of individuals are healed by attending to their body's actual needs every year.

My research and interviews indicate that this amazing lifestyle and diet can assist our bodies in healing themselves from common diseases caused by following unhealthy lifestyle, as listed below. The degree of healing depends on the extent of the damage imposed on the body.

• Cardiovascular diseases
• Cancer (with proper nutrition and lifestyle changes shown to reduce risk, support the immune system, and in some cases improve outcomes alongside treatment)
• Multiple Sclerosis (MS)
• Type 2 Diabetes
• Liver diseases such as cirrhosis and fatty liver
• Arthritis
• High blood pressure
• High levels of LDL (low-density lipoprotein) cholesterol
• Migraine
• Constipation
• Reflux and other stomach conditions

This list is merely an example, and typically, you may not even catch a cold or get headaches.

Several people were healed of so-called incurable diseases. I heard about people who improved dramatically from psoriasis by going fully Raw Vegan. Psoriasis is considered a chronic, long-term inflammatory skin condition with no conventional cure.

Another woman reported recovery from endometriosis, also classified as incurable, a chronic condition that can affect long-term health.

You may need fasting for a quicker healing process. Some of the masters of the Raw Vegan (Raw Fruitarian) diet introduce a 21-day (or even longer) water fast for people with advanced or more challenging conditions. Mono-fruit fasting, such as grape or orange fasting, is another approach that has been used to expedite the healing process in some cases.

Often, doctors describe the healing process as miraculous when patients survive against all odds. When discussing someone who has healed from a chronic or "incurable" disease by adopting a fully Raw Vegan (Raw Fruitarian) diet, health practitioners' reactions may vary from denial to attributing it to chance.

Anne Osborne, the author of "Fruitarianism: The Path to Paradise," who resides in Queensland, Australia, is one example. She chose the natural path primarily for the health and vitality it offered. From her early childhood, she had a compassionate feeling for animals. When she turned 18, she learned about veganism and the potential health benefits and increased compassion for animals it could bring.

She gave it a try and was amazed by the immediate results. Remembering her school on the hills, getting there had often been a challenge for her. After becoming vegan, her energy improved noticeably, and walking up those hills became much easier. This was one of the first clear results of changing her diet. It challenged the common belief that meat is the best source of energy and strength.

About two years later, she attended a brief talk above a bar by a local author, David Shelley, about Fruitarianism. Loving the talk, she found David's book inspiring and began a fruitarian journey that persists to this day. She has experimented with mono-fruit diets, such as 21 days on grapes or even six months on melons only. After more than 30 years of being fully Raw Fruitarian, she continues to enjoy excellent health, abundant energy, and a life free from diseases or medications.

She also raised her children fully Raw Fruitarian, and both are healthy, respectful to plants and animals and have had none of the common childhood illnesses despite close contact with other children suffering from them. She believes a natural, healthy, and holistic life combines a correct diet, exercise, sunshine, enough rest, and fresh air daily. Her message is clear: do your research, increase your knowledge, prepare emotionally, mentally, and spiritually, and then act with faith. In her words, you will enjoy a healthy lifestyle for life. You can find more about Anne's experience and lifestyle in her website: https://fruitgod.com/

Anne is an example of someone who chose this path primarily to improve her health condition. However, for many people who adopt a natural lifestyle on a Raw Vegan (Raw Fruitarian) diet, their journey begins because they have been severely ill and traditional medical treatments or pharmaceuticals didn't offer them a real cure. Some have faced conditions such as cancer, diabetes, multiple sclerosis, and other aggressive or "incurable" diseases.

When conventional medicine could not provide relief, they turned; often as a last resort; to a fully Raw Vegan (Raw Fruitarian) diet. For many, this shift gave their bodies the conditions they needed to begin healing[1].

---

[1] This path may not heal all diseases, depending on the type and the advancement of the disease.

I was amazed to hear that several women reported little to no menstrual bleeding after adopting a Raw Vegan lifestyle, yet still experienced normal ovulation and gave birth to healthy babies. I don't think health science can fully explain this yet, and I couldn't find proper research about this fascinating outcome. While peer-reviewed studies directly linking Raw Vegan diets to reduced menstrual bleeding are limited, there is emerging research showing that plant-based diets can influence hormonal balance, inflammation, and cycle regularity. These mechanisms may help explain some of the observations people report, though more studies are needed.

There are also individuals with serious conditions such as diabetes and cancer who have reported improvements by following a natural diet and aligning with their body's real needs. Others with less recognised and traditionally considered "incurable" conditions, such as epilepsy and endometriosis, have also described healing when nourished exclusively with Raw Vegan food.

Now, many of these people strongly advocate for natural living, raise awareness about the importance of respecting the body, and share their experiences to inspire others. Here are some of the voices from this growing community who would love to share their stories.

D. Hope N. from Arizona- USA

At the young age of 32, Hope was diagnosed with Fibromyalgia[1]. Her doctors suggested it might be genetic and prescribed

---

[1] Fibromyalgia is a chronic disorder characterised by widespread musculoskeletal pain, fatigue, and tenderness in localised areas. (see Glossary)

medications, warning that without them she could end up in a wheelchair.

She was also suffering from shingles[1] and severe Asthma[2], which once became so critical that she required intensive care. Despite these challenges, Hope did not lose her hope and was searching for a proper solution for her condition to get back to her total health. She always wanted to be a strong and supportive mom for her 2-year-old daughter. She got some assistance and did water physical therapy after being bed-bound for months.

One day, when she was watching TV, a show called "Extreme Diets" started, and part of it was explaining the Raw Vegan diet and its results. The following day, she decided to test the Raw Vegan and went fully Raw.

It only took a little time before the fantastic results were revealed. After several months of detoxification, Hope returned to her Ultimate Health. She got back on her feet with no assistance, and not only could she walk again, but running became one of her everyday activities. Imagine the joy of going from being confined to bed for months to running freely in the park!

Her asthma and shingles resolved, and she reached her healthy weight by shedding about 120 lbs (54 kg) in just six months. Her eyesight also improved, and she began wearing slimmer glasses. I was amazed when I saw her before-and-after Raw Vegan photos; the transformation was astounding.

She took an age test after a few years of being a Raw Vegan and was surprised to see that she was at least 11 years younger than her chronological age. The examiner stated that their test findings are

---

[1] Shingles, also known as herpes zoster, is a viral infection that causes a painful rash. (see Glossary)

[2] Asthma is a chronic respiratory condition characterised by inflammation and narrowing of the airways, which can cause difficulty in breathing. (see Glossary)

frequently in the opposite direction and that people have a higher biological age than their chronological one!

Hope is now enjoying her beautiful life with her family, and her message is: "Stop using time and money as an excuse to be unhealthy; if you have the time and money to live on fast food, you have the time and the money to eat nutrient-rich Raw foods."

Anil Nagpal- Mumbai- India

Another person who transformed his health by adopting Raw Veganism is Anil.

Like many children, he had health challenges early in life. Doctors surgically removed his tonsils after repeated infections and sore throats.

As he grew older, his health continued to be compromised. He struggled with high cholesterol and sleep disorders, which required medication. At the age of 43, he was diagnosed with type 2 diabetes. His fasting blood sugar was 310 mg/dL, and doctors prescribed him 2 mg of blood sugar control tablets daily.

Over the next ten years, his dosage gradually escalated to 2000 mg per day with different types of medication. During this time, he also developed kidney stones and hypertension.

Seeking a real solution, he attended multiple health seminars, but most only emphasised medication and disease management. In 2016, he finally heard a speaker discuss the benefits of a Raw Vegan lifestyle for human health. After further research, he began his Raw Vegan journey, and within four months, he stopped all medications, including those for diabetes.

His blood sugar dropped to a normal fasting range of 90 mg/dL, and he reported energy levels that felt 25 years younger. He also lost 24 kg, dropping from 74 to 50 kg, reaching his ideal weight.

Anil later took a biological age test, and the result showed he was 15 years younger than his chronological age. He also noticed a positive emotional shift: his anger subsided, and he felt calmer with his new lifestyle. He firmly believes that body and mind are deeply connected, and a healthy body creates the foundation for a healthy mind.

Now, at 57, Anil is happily living with his family, enjoying what he describes as an "ever-young" feeling. His message is: "People often focus only on survival. It is essential to learn how to live fully, without constant health problems or endless doctor visits."

He remains grateful to his family, his Raw Vegan community, and his supportive vegan doctors for their encouragement during his transformation.

Janette Murray-Wakelin – QLD Australia

Janette has a fantastic story to share.

Janette, who is the author of two books: 'Raw Can Cure Cancer' and 'Running Out of Time-Running Raw Around Australia' and a co-star in the internationally acclaimed film 'RAW the Documentary' is the world record holder of 366 consecutive marathons running while being Raw Vegan all around Australia!

This is amazing, isn't it? I could not imagine someone could run a marathon every single day all year around and be fully Raw Vegan.

Here is a brief of her story.

In 2001, she was diagnosed with highly aggressive carcinoma breast cancer, and she was given only six months to live.

The tumour was 3 cm, and the cancer had spread to the chest wall and the lymph nodes. She was shocked by the diagnosis as she has always been highly active in her life and thought she had a fantastic diet, being a vegan for the last 15 years and vegetarian for the previous 25 years. She had never been sick in her life and had never taken any medicines, not even an aspirin! The doctors recommended conventional chemotherapy and radiation treatment, which might extend her life a further six months.

At 52 years old, a mother of two and grandmother of one, she was unwilling to accept this prognosis. The power of her intention was far greater than her fear, and she was determined to stay around for a longer time. Her intuitive response to the recommended treatment was not to compromise the body's defense system further. Instead, she should help her body rejuvenate and rebuild itself.

Her instinct told her treating the symptoms would not address the cause, and she took the diagnosis as a challenge. She extensively researched the cause, recommended treatments, and holistic therapies for the disease. With the help of her naturopathic physician, she increased her oxygen intake. She boosted her immune system by eating 100% Raw and natural living foods and increasing her daily exercises, yoga and running. Only 6 months after her diagnosis, she received a clean bill of health. There was no longer any sign of cancer cells in her body.

She finished the therapy regime but has continued with all other aspects of her Raw lifestyle. After 23 years, she is disease-free and enjoys a great, healthy life. With the help of her husband, Janette established a Centre of Optimum Health and now offers Personalised Raw Vegan Conscious Health Retreats from their home in Queensland Australia to help others achieve their Ultimate Health.

Janette is an excellent example of someone who believed she always had a healthy lifestyle and was amazed to experience the difference of changing her life from eating cooked food to a new world of energy, mind clarity and healing of eating Raw.

Her message is: "There is no better time to change to a healthy Raw Vegan diet than now. Our responsibility is to make conscious lifestyle choices for the health of all living beings, future generations, and the planet's health. We are never too young and certainly never too old to make a change that can make a difference. The most important thing to remember is that we are worth it. Don't wait for the diagnosis; make the change now!"

I was truly amazed by interviewing her and reading her entire story at her website: https://Rawveganpath.com

Hope, Anil, and Janette are just a few examples of people who have experienced remarkable improvements after embracing a Raw Vegan lifestyle. I interviewed them and shared their stories here to inspire you to take steps toward this path and enjoy your complete and Ultimate Health for the rest of your life.

It is important to remember, however, that a healed body can slip back into its old state if someone returns to their previous diet and reintroduces harmful substances, especially in large quantities. If you want to maintain a full, healthy life after overcoming sickness, staying on the path of a natural lifestyle is usually essential.

I would like to mention that lifestyle and diet changes are widely recognised as effective in improving many chronic conditions, such as type 2 diabetes, cardiovascular disease, high cholesterol, and obesity. Plant-based diets have also been shown to support better immune function, reduce inflammation, and improve quality of life for people with autoimmune and inflammatory conditions. While there is encouraging evidence for plant-based approaches in cancer care and other complex diseases, more research is still needed. Importantly, such lifestyle changes should ideally be made under medical supervision, especially when reducing or stopping prescribed drugs, to ensure safety and proper monitoring.

Energy Level

Tony Robbins[1] says: "Life is Energy!"

Our level of happiness has a direct relationship with our level of energy. Have you ever noticed that you would feel good when you go to nature? The energy of living things; trees, plants, even animals can uplift us and restore balance. You also may wonder why people keep plants and pets at home.

Energy influences everything. When we feel energised our organs work well and we are at a higher level of thinking and mental health. A higher level of energy can also help us connect to a deeper sense of spirituality.

Life always brings challenges and handling them requires resilience. In difficult moments, having more energy helps us feel less stressed and respond with a clearer, calmer mind. People often search for ways to lift their level of energy. For example, some

---

[1] Anthony Jay Robbins is an American author, coach, and a well-known motivation speaker.

turn to alcohol, which can stimulate blood flow and create a temporary feeling of euphoria.

If you have tried it, you may recall that alcohol gives only a short-lived boost. Once the effect wears off, you can feel drained, sometimes for days. This often leads people to reach for alcohol again, chasing the same lift, though it never lasts. And along the way come the side effects: headaches, mood swings, poor sleep, even dependency.

In fact, alcohol is well recognised as a toxin that can cause harm in both the short and long term, depending on the dose and frequency of use. Scientifically, alcohol is broken down in the liver into acetaldehyde, a compound even more toxic than alcohol itself. Acetaldehyde triggers oxidative stress, damages cells, and depletes antioxidants that normally protect us. This is one reason why "hangover symptoms" such as fatigue, nausea, or foggy thinking appear the next day. Over time, repeated use burdens the liver and other organs, which is why long-term drinking is linked to liver disease and accelerated aging.

Now you may ask, with all these side effects, why do some people still turn to alcohol? Isn't the answer simply the lure of a short burst of energy and the temporary feeling of being good?

Coffee and tea are the other ones. Let's talk about coffee. You might have seen that coffee beans are green when they are harvested. Then the industry roasts them with high temperature and makes them completely brown, close to black colour. Roasting changes their chemistry by triggering the Maillard reaction and **caramelisation**, creating hundreds of new compounds. This process also alters the taste; for example, chlorogenic acids break down into quinic and caffeic acids, making coffee more **bitter**.

Alongside the flavour change, the chemistry also creates stimulation. Roasting releases and modifies caffeine-related compounds and other biologically active substances.

But stimulation is not the whole story. Roasting also places stress on the body by generating byproducts such as acrylamide and polycyclic aromatic hydrocarbons (PAHs), especially at high roast levels. These are considered undesirable.

While darker roasting can increase stimulation, it also reduces some of the natural antioxidants in coffee beans and leaves behind a greater load of unwanted byproducts. In short, the darker the roast, the stronger the kick; but also the heavier the chemical burden your body must process.

Although scientific research does show some benefits of coffee, once you've cleaned your body of toxins and returned it to its natural state, you may be surprised by how even a few drops of coffee affect you. What once felt harmless can suddenly bring discomfort, showing how sensitive a healthy body is to unnecessary stimulants. Despite its popularity, coffee still carries compounds created during roasting that can place stress on the body; particularly when your system is already functioning at its best.

Tea is almost the same. Fresh tea leaves are naturally rich in antioxidants, especially catechins. But when the leaves are fermented and heavily oxidised to make black tea, many of these antioxidants are reduced or altered. Green tea, being less processed, usually keeps more of its beneficial compounds.

While tea still contains helpful polyphenols, the stronger the processing, the fewer protective antioxidants remain. Like coffee, tea gives stimulation; but it also comes with changes in chemistry that the body must handle.

Please note that when we introduce certain stimulating substances into the body, it responds by directing more blood to the digestive system to help process and eliminate them. This temporarily increases **metabolism** (the body's internal burning process). As a result, our energy level may rise, and we feel a short-term lift.

However, these substances can also influence the brain and nervous system, sometimes dulling or numbing signals depending on the dose. This is one reason people may not feel the usual "hunger signals" from their cells for a time. Yet our genuine, healthy cells (not the compromised ones) always require genuine nourishment from natural food, not heavily processed or oxidised versions. They are constantly sending signals when they need fuel; and real food is the only way to answer them properly.

I'm often surprised when I come across articles, even from scientific sources, that promote the supposed benefits of alcohol or coffee. For example, I once read a piece claiming that coffee could help with fat burning. While there may be some truth to this, it is only one side of the story. What about the byproducts in coffee that can overstimulate the nervous system and place stress on the brain? And what about the increased risk of cardiovascular strain, including heart attack, linked to high consumption? Is coffee really the only way to support fat loss? If that were the case, wouldn't all heavy coffee drinkers be slim and full of health? Clearly, that is not what we see.

To understand the issue with stimulation, think of the economy. Governments usually offer stimulus only during a crisis, to help lift things temporarily. Stimulation is never meant to be permanent. No wise government would continue a stimulus budget for the long term, because the economy would eventually overheat and spiral out of control.

In the same way, many people push their bodies into constant stimulation instead of allowing recovery. Without real nourishment from whole foods, they become reliant on these temporary boosts, which may feel good in the moment but carry long-term costs. Think of someone who cannot start their day without two strong coffees or an energy drink just to function; the body is running on borrowed energy, not genuine vitality.

Alcohol, another example, can put extra strain on the liver. Over time this can reduce the liver's ability to produce antioxidants, weakening one of the body's key defenses against cellular damage. When this balance is lost, the effects often show up on the skin, especially on the face, which is very sensitive to internal changes. In fact, the body sometimes uses the skin as an emergency outlet when the main detox pathways, like the digestive system, are overloaded.

You may have noticed how quickly people, especially women, show signs of aging in their skin when poor dietary choices and alcohol consumption become regular habits. Over time, the skin loses its natural glow, elasticity, and clarity. In response, many turn to skincare or beauty products in hopes of reversing the process. While some products may provide some improvements, many are ultimately limited in effect, and some can even cause additional strain on the skin.

From my perspective, alcohol, coffee, cigarettes, drugs, energy drinks, and even some prescribed medicines share a common thread. They may provide short-term boosts of energy or relief, but the long-term price is often damage to vital organs. Recognising this difference between **temporary stimulation** and genuine nourishment is key to protecting both your health and your natural appearance.

I hope I could explain the issues with stimulators and their side effects. Now let us get back to our energy level with a proper diet. At a young age, we are full of energy because the effects of cooked and unhealthy food and drinks have not fully shown themselves yet. Our organs are young, and our bodies can process these challenges more efficiently. Also, young kids usually introduce fewer stimulants to their bodies than adults; for example, they don't drink coffee or alcohol. Children's energy is also naturally higher due to their faster metabolism and growth.

We talked about the energy we need to be functional. We also talked about how energy gets created, and when we eat heavily cooked or processed food, it is harder for the body to digest and convert into clean energy. When we consume Raw materials, we allow ourselves to digest them more easily and access energy more directly; alcohol or other stimulation is no longer necessary, and you will notice how your skin naturally regains its brightness.

In addition, our digestive system expends a significant amount of energy to function. Generally, raw materials require much less time to be digested. For instance, fruits typically spend only 2–4 hours in the central part of the digestive system, while many green leafy vegetables take 4–6 hours, and activated nuts may require up to 6–8 hours. In contrast, the digestion of many high temp cooked or processed foods may take as long as 24 hours. This extended duration is often due to the greater effort required to break down altered or heavily processed structures, leading to increased strain on the body as it works diligently.

I know some individuals who experienced constipation lasting over three days. This means the food stays in their digestive system over 72 hours and uses much more energy. When food stays too long in the body, it can ferment and put stress on the gut, encouraging the growth of harmful bacteria and viruses, which pressure the immune system and drain even more energy.

When the digestive system malfunctions, nutrient absorption is distorted, resulting in inadequate intake of necessary substances, including minerals and vitamins. How many people do you know with digestive issues? I was one of them when I was ignorant, eating burnt food all the time.

These are a few examples of how we lose our energy daily and try to compensate for it by stimulation, long sleeping, and doing activities such as gaming, which pumps adrenaline, another stimulator.

The natural way is different. By eating Raw living foods and allowing your body to detox, you gradually and sustainably raise your energy level. This boost is not artificial, and unlike alcohol or coffee, it does not cause other issues to the body.

When you live naturally, your sleep quality often improves, and you may find you need less sleep than before. You'll experience deep, restorative rest each night and wake up feeling fully energised, much like when you were a child.

When your digestive system functions optimally, your body's cells don't need to keep signalling hunger for real nourishment. Instead, you feel calm, balanced, and supported by a steady energy supply that comes from living in harmony with your natural design.

Fitness

"You are Made of whatever you Intake!"

Who does not believe that being overweight is one of humanity's most significant health challenges in recent decades? Excess weight often develops from eating the wrong foods and not exercising enough. However, food is usually the primary driver of obesity.

A lot of research (see References) indicates that obesity is a primary risk factor for various diseases, including cardiovascular disease, diabetes, osteoarthritis, and more. Still, obesity itself is better understood not as a disease, but as a symptom of an unhealthy lifestyle, often shaped by poor dietary habits. It's important to note that in some cases, hormonal imbalances such as thyroid dysfunction contribute to weight gain. These imbalances can be aggravated by an overload of unwanted compounds in the body, particularly in glands like the thyroid, as well as a lack of essential nutrients such as iodine, which is critical for thyroid hormone production.

I've seen TV programs claim that lack of exercise leads to weight gain. Conversely, I've also seen programs suggesting exercise for weight gain. Confusing, isn't it?

The fact is that **regular physical activity is essential** for our health. As I mentioned earlier, the lymphatic system does not have a pump and relies on body movement to function effectively. Exercise also boosts metabolism, which helps burn stored fat and improves the body's detoxification capacity by enhancing the activity of internal organs.

That said, diet usually has the greatest influence on long-term health. Some professional athletes still get sick if they eat junk food, while I've also met people who rarely exercise but maintain good health because they consistently choose proper food.

There are many diets and weight loss systems on the market aiming to help people address their overweight issues and health complications due to obesity. While these systems may work to some degree, most of them provide only temporary solutions, as people often find them difficult to sustain. Additionally, some lack a proper theoretical foundation and may not make sense to follow in a long run.

With a natural lifestyle, people often shed excess weight naturally if they are overweight. For example, I know someone who dropped from 145 kg to 70 kg in less than six months simply by following one clear principle: eating *Raw Vegan foods*.

Those who commit to a natural lifestyle usually reach their ideal weight within the first three to six months. This is remarkable, isn't it? Let's look at why this happens so quickly.

We've already discussed how unwanted compounds can accumulate in the body and how it manages them. In addition to its detoxification systems, the body uses two main defence strategies: producing extra fat cells and diluting the harmful load in fluids.

Soft tissues, particularly fat cells, are prime storage areas. While fat naturally serves as an energy reserve, when the body is overloaded, it creates more fat cells specifically to store harmful substances.

Another strategy is dilution. By holding water around these substances, the body weakens their impact and shields sensitive organs. This is one reason people on the Typical Western Diet (T.W.D.) are advised to drink large amounts of water; often around 2.5 litres per day. Much of this water is retained to buffer the effects of poor food intake. You may have noticed how thirsty you get after a salty meal or a greasy burger; that thirst is your body asking for help to dilute what it can't process easily.

When we cease or reduce the intake of **harmful compounds** into our bodies, accumulated ones begin to circulate within the bloodstream for elimination. By maintaining a natural lifestyle, toxin levels decrease, and our body no longer needs to retain excess fat cells and stored water. Consequently, significant weight loss occurs, primarily from the reduction of fat and water stored between tissues. Without the necessity of toxin accumulation, the body naturally returns to its original, nature-designed shape.

During the first two weeks of a Raw diet, individuals may observe darker urine. This change in urine color is often indicative of the rapid elimination of those harmful substances, characterised by their distinct and sometimes unpleasant odor, through the digestive system. Millions of body cells undergo natural turnover daily, being replaced by new cells generated by our body's organs. My research indicates that the quality of those new cells depends on the raw materials you provide. A diet rich in fresh, nutrient-dense foods supplies antioxidants, vitamins, and minerals that support strong, resilient cells. On the other hand, diets heavy in processed or heat damaged foods provide fewer protective nutrients and more oxidative stress, which can make cells more vulnerable to malfunction.

Think of it this way: your body is constantly "rebuilding" itself. Give it the right building blocks and it creates solid, healthy structures. Feed it weak or damaged building blocks, and the new structures are compromised. Over time, this difference shows up in your energy, your immunity, your skin, and even your risk of chronic disease

It's also common to experience cravings when first moving away from cooked or processed foods. This mainly changes in your brain chemistry, taste preferences, and even gut microbiota adjusting to a new fuel source.

With consistency, these cravings fade, your palate resets, and your body thrives on the nourishment it was designed for.

Most Raw Vegans find themselves skinny at the start of their journey, especially in the first year as they lose their weaker cells. But this is temporary as by continuing the natural lifestyle and taking proper fuel, healthier cells gradually replace weaker ones, and as a result, the body naturally moves back toward its ideal weight. Many reported feelings rejuvenated, experiencing a surge in energy levels, and feeling as if they've regained years of vitality with their newfound genuine and healthy cells.

One of the main body parts influenced by our lifestyle is the skin, which is also the most visibly impacted. As the largest organ in the body, it is highly sensitive and often reflects our internal health. The appearance of the skin can even offer clues about a person's age.

Our skin, especially our face, plays a huge role in shaping first impressions. No one can ignore its importance for our sense of beauty and confidence. The elimination of stored waste combined with the abundant vitamins, minerals, and antioxidants in raw foods can have a powerful effect on the skin's clarity and radiance.

Have you ever noticed how soft and **wrinkle-free** children's skin is? That freshness is largely because they have not yet accumulated the same build-up of internal waste that many adults carry. Compare this to adults who often use heavy makeup to cover imperfections. You've likely seen photos of celebrities without makeup and noticed the striking difference.

By adopting a natural lifestyle, many people experience skin that looks healthier, smoother, and more youthful, often reducing the need for makeup and cosmetic treatments. The change can bring a deep sense of rejuvenation and self-confidence, as the reflection in the mirror begins to align with how vibrant they feel inside.

Scientifically skin health is closely tied to diet, hydration, and overall lifestyle. Antioxidants such as vitamin C and E, found abundantly in fruits and vegetables, help protect against oxidative stress that contributes to wrinkles and dullness. Hydration supports elasticity, while a healthy liver and digestive system help prevent breakouts and puffiness. Although no single food can guarantee perfect skin, a nutrient-rich, natural diet combined with proper rest and fresh air can make a noticeable difference in skin radiance.

Another vital organ that greatly benefits from embracing a natural lifestyle is our **eyes**. Essential nutrients such as **Vitamin A, Vitamin C, lutein, and zeaxanthin** play a significant role in maintaining healthy eyesight. By adhering to a natural way of living and consuming ample raw fruits and vegetables daily, we ensure an adequate intake of these essential vitamins and phytonutrients. Additionally, a healthy gut facilitates the proper absorption of these nutrients into our system.

Poor dietary habits, on the other hand, often go hand in hand with constipation, which we've already discussed as a sign of digestive strain. Constipation doesn't just affect the bowels; it interferes with nutrient absorption. And the eyes are among the most vulnerable organs affected by nutrient deficiencies. Individuals suffering from **constipation** often experience weakened eyesight and may require corrective eyewear.

However, by adopting a fully Raw diet rich in essential vitamins and minerals, the eyes can regain their sparkle and appear beautiful and healthy. Some individuals have even been able to discard their glasses after adhering to their natural diet.

I've often found that by observing a person's eyes and face without makeup, I can get a fairly accurate impression of their internal health. The eyes, in particular, can be like windows, reflecting the vitality of the whole body.

Living fully Raw not only supports healthy eyesight but also helps you maintain your ideal weight without the stress of complicated diets or programs. A flat stomach, glowing skin and eyes, and steady energy become natural outcomes of eating the right foods. Even your daily fitness routines become easier with this boost of vitality.

What are your fitness expectations? A toned body? A radiant face? The energy to enjoy every activity without fatigue? A Raw lifestyle can offer all of these, naturally and sustainably.

Feeling

Let me ask you a question: What would be your feelings if you were always fit, ate tasty and healthy foods and had a top energy level? Wouldn't it be amazing? You may think "oh my feeling is great!", but wait a minute, the best time to gauge your genuine feelings is immediately after you wake up on a Monday morning!

With a natural lifestyle, you consistently feel good, regardless of whether it's a Friday evening or a Monday morning. Your digestive system functions optimally, and you may experience minimal health complications. Your energy levels soar, and you find yourself needing no more sleep than necessary.

You may find that you no longer need perfumes to mask unpleasant odours, which can result from waste building up in the body. Similarly, you may notice improvements in the freshness of your breath, particularly upon waking up in the morning. Modern science also shows that foods like garlic, alcohol, and coffee release strong-smelling compounds through sweat and breath, while fruits and vegetables provide antioxidants that protect the skin and make sweat almost odourless. A clean, well-nourished body shows itself in clearer skin, fresher breath, and lighter sweat.

After years of adhering to a Raw diet, as your body detoxifies, you may find that your sweat resembles water with **minimal odour**. These days, I go to the gym almost every weekday, and my sweat nearly soaks my clothes. Years ago, when I was a vegetarian, I had to wash my sports clothes after every activity. However, these days I leave them to get dry and still can wear them the following day. I mostly wash them once a week after four or five gym sessions and still cannot smell the bad odour from them.

Experience self-love, free from the fear of diseases. In my conversations with many individuals, particularly those in middle age, their greatest concern often revolves around losing their youthful appearance. How would they feel if they knew they could maintain their beauty for much longer, or even throughout their entire lives, without fear?

The feeling is everything. We all would love to have a good living and enjoy our lives. But how can you find a sense of well-being in someone who is unwell? Many individuals spend a significant amount of funds for a unique experience and get a good feeling for a short period. We travel globally for the same purpose, good feeling! I know people get sick frequently, especially when they are travelling, and often, it ruins their travel and their purpose of feeling good. You may have heard of the Law of Attraction, which suggests that positive feelings attract good things into our lives.

A proper and balanced diet, which gives you a good feeling in your physical body, can also attract good things into your life. Consider this for a moment: Imagine a life where you're always fit, high energy level, free from health complications, and full of hope for a long and healthy future. How would you feel with such abundance in your life?

Enjoy this profound outcome after going with your natural lifestyle! And please don't forget to share your experience with me on my website.

Saving Earth

Last but certainly not least, an important outcome is the positive impact on our environment. Let's consider how a natural lifestyle benefits the health of our planet. We've previously discussed how this lifestyle benefits humans while causing less harm to other creatures. Now, let's explore the ways in which following a natural lifestyle can contribute to the well-being of our beautiful planet Earth.

You may have heard about climate change and its profound impact on our lives and the well-being of future generations. Studies (see References) suggest that one of the primary contributors to global warming is methane gas emitted from the stomachs of cows. When individuals embrace a natural lifestyle and transition to becoming Raw Vegans, the need for breeding cattle drops significantly.

This shift allows cows to return to living in harmony with nature, as they once did before the meat industry dominated our lives.

I recall seeing a study on TV showing that if even one-third of the world's population became vegan, climate change would no longer be the same threat. Imagine what could happen if that population became Raw Vegan!

It is estimated that 25 kilograms of plant food (or around 7 kg if it's grains) are required to produce just 1 kg of beef. You can picture the enormous strain this places on Earth's resources. The same holds true for sheep. In fact, in Australia alone, the sheep population is roughly double the entire human population!

Water use is another critical factor. Producing 1 kg of beef requires around 50,000 litres of water, compared to 1,000 litres for wheat, or almost none for fruit trees once they are well established in rain-rich areas. Unlike industrial farming, which relies heavily on irrigation, many fruit trees thrive with natural rainfall.

Pollution adds another layer of concern. Industrial agriculture contributes to land, air, and water contamination, weakening ecosystems worldwide. On top of this, when we cook our food, we burn fuel. By avoiding hot plates and ovens, we reduce our reliance on natural gas and electricity, cutting our carbon footprint even further.

Now, picture this: if a significant portion of the population embraced a natural lifestyle, the demand for junk products and the factories that process them would fall sharply. This would save vast amounts of energy, water, and land. And most importantly, give our planet space to breathe and **regenerate**.

The natural lifestyle is built around eating mainly fruits, leafy greens, small amounts of nuts (which come from trees), and some supplements if needed. When 80 to 90 percent of your food comes from fruit; primarily growing on trees; the agriculture industry must shift significantly toward planting fruit orchards.

This change begins to reverse the destruction of Earth's environment. Many people think of deforestation only in terms of homes and buildings, but much of it is actually linked to animal farming and large-scale cereal and vegetable cultivation.

Trees are vital allies in climate balance. They capture CO_2; the main gas driving global warming; and in return, they provide oxygen, our most precious element. Yes, they release small amounts of CO_2 at night, but their daytime oxygen production far outweighs it. In short, trees are net oxygen producers, true companions of life.

Organic fruit trees do not require harmful chemicals, another aspect of minimising environmental damage. Trees also supply food and nutrition for other creatures, which are part of the essential biodiversity and our beautiful environment. Consider how the removal of jungles impacts the lives of humans, other animals, and small creatures.

Healthy soil is another benefit of fruit tree farming. Soil thrives when left undisturbed. Orchards protect the delicate topsoil and its living community of microbes, fungi, and small creatures. Unlike intensive animal farming or ploughed vegetable fields, fruit trees allow these vital organisms to flourish. This strengthens the soil and sustains long-term fertility.

Now, imagine stepping outside and finding fruit trees in every neighbourhood, providing food, beauty, and shade. Do your own research and ask yourself: what harm can a fruit tree do to Earth, and what benefits can it bring instead?

On a personal level, the main "waste" of this lifestyle is fruit and vegetable scraps which can be composted and used to fertilise gardens. A Raw Vegan may not need freezers full of processed food or stacks of canned goods. This means fewer plastics, less packaging, and more savings for the environment and your wallet!

When I first became vegetarian, few people understood the concept. Friends would sometimes offer me chicken, thinking it didn't count as meat.

Twenty years ago, very few people worldwide were aware of the vegan diet. Now, it has become a major trend, with thousands of articles about its benefits being published every day. The natural life style by embracing Raw diet, hailed as the ultimate solution for human health, is poised to become increasingly popular.

As more individuals experience its benefits, they will spread the word. In the years to come, together, we can not only enhance human health but also protect our beautiful planet Earth, its wonderful animals, and all its creatures.

Picture this: walking through your neighbourhood and seeing fruit trees on every corner, children picking fresh food straight from nature, families living with health and vitality, animals roaming freely, and clean air filling your lungs. No heavy pollution, no excess packaging, no overworked land; just harmony between people and the Earth.

This is the world that embracing a Raw Vegan lifestyle can help create. Not only a healthier body for ourselves, but a healthier, brighter, and more sustainable future for all living beings.

This is my dream; and I believe it is not far from becoming reality.

Quick Favour?

If *Health on Fire* has been helpful or insightful for you, I'd be so grateful if you could take a moment to leave an **honest, unbiased review**. Your feedback not only supports my work but also helps others who may need this message discover the book.

Grab the **Quick Guide to the Raw Diet + 7-Day Raw Meal Plan**; normally a $199 resource, but **Free** for all readers. Email your proof of purchase to info@michaelzara.com.au with the subject **"Reader Bonus – Health on Fire"** and you will receive a copy!

You can leave a quick review on

Amazon: https://www.amazon.com/dp/B0DNK3JW87

Goodreads:https://www.goodreads.com/book/show/221406164-health-on-fire

Thanks for supporting my work! — **Michael Zara**

Capture 9

My Story

L ife is amazing! We grow and learn to improve our lives in every aspect. Health plays the most significant role in our journey.

A sick physical body is not a suitable vehicle for our wonderful soul to continue its advancement. It may take us to a different destination. Just as you wouldn't have a pleasant journey driving an unreliable and damaged car, a healthy body is essential for a fulfilling life. Let me share part of my journey with you.

Early Childhood

I did not have an enjoyable childhood. Like many other kids, I struggled with several health complications, mainly constipation, infections, severe headaches, and high fevers. I remember multiple occasions when my body temperature went over 41.5 °C (106.7 °F), and my parents rushed me to a specialised hospital where doctors tried various methods and medications to bring it down.

On one occasion, my fever was so persistent that it refused to drop even half a degree. A highly specialised doctor eventually injected an unfamiliar medication into my small toe, which my parents had never seen before, and it finally worked. Without that intervention, I might not be here today to write this book about health.

I remember several times I had seizures; especially during the night; and all my sweet dreams became nightmares, leaving me with very little sleep and unbearable headaches. I caught colds and flu regularly, and many times I had to undergo multiple penicillin injections, sometimes up to 12 shots of 1.2 million units over two weeks, just to recover enough to get back on my feet.

Since childhood, I have been thinking and searching for a healthier lifestyle. I saw people sick almost all the time. One of my cousins took about 20 different tablets every day, and her favourite journey seemed to be between her home, hospitals, testing laboratories, and pharmacies.

Being sick so often, and watching people around me suffer with health complications that also affected their mental state and happiness, always raised a question in my mind: If we are the most advanced creatures on Earth, why does our physiology seem so weak? Is it possible to achieve lasting health without relying so heavily on medications and treatments?

Diet Evolved

After studying a few holistic health books, my primary understanding was that "we are built from what we consume." It is like a building made from its construction materials. I realised the main source of health problems is food, particularly unhealthy or junk foods. A simple way to put it: "If we always eat junk, our body becomes junk."

Then, I started removing junk foods from my diet, including soft drinks, burgers, chips, coffee, and tea. From then on, I felt much healthier, with higher energy and fewer health complications. However, some challenges remained.

I was still catching colds, having headaches a couple of times a week, and experiencing severe migraine attacks about once a month. Sometimes, I even had to stay in the hospital for migraine treatments. I remember one occasion when I was crossing a street, and a severe migraine hit me so suddenly that I fainted for a few seconds. I was lucky to wake up lying in the middle of the road without being hit by a car and people ran towards me!

On another occasion, when I had a migraine, none of the common painkillers were effective to reduce the pain. My closest friend, who was a medical doctor, injected me with 2 ml of Ketamine, a drug used for general anaesthesia. You may not believe it, but even Ketamine did not work completely; I was still left with some pain!

The persistence of these health problems pushed me to continue researching the true sources of disease. From reading people's experiences and research (see References) by vegan scientists and organisations, I learned that one of the primary contributors to common diseases such as cancer and cardiovascular disease is meat and other animal products. At that point, I decided to test a vegetarian diet and see the results for myself.

I became a vegetarian for about 13 years. The change helped me a lot, and my health improved. Alongside being vegetarian, I kept researching and gradually stopped eating processed food. I rigorously checked product labels to ensure they did not contain artificial flavours, colours, or preservatives. I also switched to organic foods as much as possible. These changes gave me a better feeling and reduced many of my health issues; however, I still experienced problems and low energy.

I continued to suffer from high blood pressure, high cholesterol, joint pain, digestive issues, stomach pain, and reflux. Although my migraines were less frequent, occurring about once every three months, they still came back. Constipation remained common, and snoring was another issue. It was also hard for me to wake up early and feel good.

This continued until a miracle happened! In early 2017, during a short conversation with one of my teammates in our Saturday soccer team, he asked about my lifestyle and diet. I mentioned I was vegetarian, and his first question was: "Why do you cook vegetables?" Embarrassed, I couldn't find a logical answer and simply said, "Because everyone does." His response stuck with me: "Just because everyone is doing something doesn't make it right!" That sentence inspired me to research cooking itself and dig deeper.

It took me about four to five months to read several books about Raw foods, listen to Raw Vegan talks and converse with the same Raw Vegan teammate. I could not find a clear answer to that simple question: why do we introduce heat(cooking) to almost all of our foods? Struggling to find a proper response finally led me to test on a Raw Vegan diet. I discussed this with my wonderful wife, who was supportive and didn't discourage me. At the time, I thought of it only as a test.

The first two weeks were a real challenge, as I went through intensive detoxification. However, after this period, the results were unbelievable! My energy level soared to a level I had never experienced before. My health reached a standard I had been searching for over 30 years.

Here are some of the results:

- Still full of energy even after playing soccer for two hours on Saturdays.

- My weight dropped initially from 79 to 67 kg, then gradually stabilised at 70 kg; my best shape
- My blood pressure dropped from 140 /90 mmHg to 97/67 mmHg. I was suffering for decades from high blood pressure.
- High LDL (bad cholesterol) reduced
- My heartbeat dropped from 88 bpm to 61 bpm
- No more pain in my joints
- Migraine cured completely
- No headache
- No constipation or diarrhea
- Snoring is gone, and my sleeping pattern has improved
- A relaxed and empty stomach with a proper digestive system

I felt about 15 -20 years younger than my chronological age.

I want to share one of the most fascinating healings that happened to me in the fourth year of my Raw Vegan journey. From my teenage years, I started developing a black spot on the skin around the ankle of my right foot. Initially, it was small, but it gradually expanded, eventually reaching about 80 mm in diameter. Over time, the skin began peeling, and the area became very itchy.

I visited our family doctor, who diagnosed it as eczema and prescribed a cream. I used it for some time, and although it reduced the itching, the black spot remained. A couple of months later, the cream stopped working and the itching returned.

I went back to the doctor, and this time he prescribed a corticosteroid medicine (I can't recall the exact name). It managed to control the issue temporarily, but the black spot persisted. After two weeks, once I stopped using the drug, the spot became extremely itchy again; so much that it kept me awake at night.

I restarted the medication occasionally, depending on the level of pain. After a few more months, I realised that if I didn't use it, the spot would become unbearable. I went back to the doctor once again, and he advised me to stop the medicine altogether, warning me about the severe side effects of long-term use. He also told me there was no permanent cure and that I would simply have to live with the itchy black spot for the rest of my life.

I lived with this itchy, peeling skin for about 30 years; until I started my natural lifestyle. Gradually, I noticed the spot fading. Having lived with it for decades, I couldn't believe what was happening. After 30 years of pain and discomfort, my ankle was completely healed: no black area, no peeling, no itching, no pain.

Formal Study

I started researching and studying health books at a very young age to understand how our body and mind work and the best way to achieve the condition I call *Ultimate Health*.

By the time I finished high school, I had already read several books on health and psychology (my favourite subject in those days).

Because of family expectations; and as my older brothers were engineers; I was pushed to follow the same path. I went to a technical university and studied mechanical engineering. Engineering was not my natural or favourite field, but I finished and graduated as a professional mechanical engineer in 1997.

However, I didn't stop there. My curiosity about the true sources of health led me to continue informal study. I spoke with health practitioners, absorbed their knowledge, and read some books and articles they recommended. My friends who were doctors and researchers helped me understand how the body works, what medicines are, and how they interact with our physiology.

In mid-2021, I decided to formalise my knowledge and enrolled in a nutrition course with The Nutrition Institute of Australia. After about 18 months of comprehensive study, I graduated in early 2023. I also completed the advanced Plant-Based (Vegan) Diet course with the same institute, graduating with the highest mark.

I thoroughly enjoyed the courses and gained deep insights into:

- How the digestive system functions

- The interconnections between body and mind

- The essential nutrients our body needs, their daily recommended intake, and best sources

- How to interpret food labels and assess supermarket products critically

Graduating from these courses and becoming a health coach and nutrition advisor felt like an outstanding achievement. This was especially meaningful given that I was balancing being a father of three, working full time, writing this book, and maintaining a happy family life. This would not have been possible without the high energy and resilience provided by my natural lifestyle; and, of course, the support of my family.

During the last eight years of being fully Raw, I've gone through different stages of detoxification, each year feeling stronger and clearer. And my journey hasn't stopped. I still read, study, and research this amazing lifestyle to better understand our body's true needs and the root causes of the dangerous diseases so many people face today.

Just as engineering taught me to respect design, nutrition taught me to respect nature's design of the human body. When I look back, I see one truth standing tall above all else: with the right fuel, the right knowledge, and the right habits, our body is capable of miracles.

When to Eat & What Nutrition?

We have already discussed how important our lifestyle, diet, and daily intake are, and why it is crucial to honour our body's true needs instead of damaging it with the unhealthy foods. We also touched on cooking, how heat can change food and sometimes create toxins, and why minimising these toxins supports better health.

After hearing all this, you may now ask me: *what exactly should we eat to be healthy?* This is a natural and important question. For many people, change feels intimidating; especially when they have followed family traditions or social habits for years. But once you begin to see real results, the motivation to continue grows, and you'll be encouraged to do deeper research and move forward on your natural path toward **Ultimate Health**.

First, I want to make it clear that I am not a qualified dietitian who can prescribe specific meal plans. What I share here is based on my personal research, study, and lived experience.

You should always do your own research, talk to trusted health professionals, and seek their guidance; especially from practitioners who themselves follow a natural lifestyle. Their advice can help you adapt this path to your unique needs.

What I can offer you is knowledge from my years of learning, experimenting, and observing results. I hope this can serve as a starting point for your own journey; helping you explore what works best for your health, your environment, and the food available in your area.

With that in mind, let's now look at some practical insights on when to eat and what to eat to fuel your body for lasting energy and health.

When to Eat

From my research and experience, our body seems to move through **three natural daily cycles**, each lasting around eight hours:

- **Cycle One (4 a.m. – 12 p.m.) – Elimination**
  This is when the body is focused on cleansing and removing waste. Many natural health traditions suggest avoiding heavy meals in this window so the body can prioritise elimination. Instead, hydration with water and fresh, juicy fruits can support this process. Circadian biology research shows that metabolism and digestive enzyme activity are **slower in the early morning** and peak around midday. This means the body is naturally less efficient at handling large, heavy meals early in the day. Studies also show that overnight fasting supports gut repair, detoxification, and immune function. By keeping mornings lighter, you align with your body's natural rhythms and give it the best chance to complete its nightly clean-up process. Regular morning bowel movements are one of the clearest signs of a healthy body, as eliminating waste daily in the morning reflects a well-functioning digestive system.

- **Cycle Two (12 p.m. – 8 p.m.) – Digestion**
  This is the ideal time to eat your main meals. Our digestive fire is strongest in the middle of the day, which aligns with scientific studies showing digestive enzyme activity, stomach acid secretion, and insulin sensitivity peak during the middle of the day. This is why many researchers recommend placing the largest meal between late morning and mid-afternoon. Studies in chrononutrition show that eating in sync with daylight hours improves glucose control and reduces the risk of metabolic disease. Heavier foods like bananas, papaya, figs, dates, if desired, greens, salads nuts, or seeds are best digested during this window.

- **Cycle Three (8 p.m. – 4 a.m.) – Assimilation & Rest**
  Here, the body is focused on absorbing nutrients and repairing itself. Eating heavy meals late at night can interfere with both processes, which is why modern sleep and metabolic research strongly recommends lighter dinners and avoiding food close to bedtime. At night, melatonin levels rise, and metabolism slows, shifting the body's focus to tissue repair, immune activity, and memory consolidation. Late-night eating is associated with poorer nutrient absorption, weight gain, and disturbed circadian rhythms. Fasting during this period supports gut rest, improved metabolic health, and deeper sleep quality.

While this "three-cycle model" comes from holistic health teachings rather than mainstream physiology, it harmonises with what circadian biology tells us: the body has natural rhythms for digestion, elimination, and repair. By syncing our eating habits with these rhythms, we allow the body to work with ease rather than under stress.

People on the Typical Western Diet (T.W.D.) often organise their days around breakfast, lunch, and dinner, with snacks in between.

For many, the morning starts with coffee, tea, baked goods, or fried foods. While these may provide a quick lift, by midday people can feel drowsy, low on energy, or even anxious; often without realising how much those choices play a role.

Intermittent fasting has become popular in recent years, typically involving 16 hours of fasting followed by an 8-hour eating window. Many people notice benefits, and it makes sense: giving the body a longer break from eating allows it time to rest and detoxify, while also avoiding the heavy morning meals that can weigh the system down.

The challenge comes when the eating window is filled with highly processed or nutrient-poor foods. Without the right fuel, the body may struggle over time, leading to fatigue, nutritional gaps, and eventually frustration; which is why some people give up.

From my experience, we don't need to lock ourselves into rigid labels of "breakfast, lunch, and dinner." When living more naturally, the body begins to send genuine signals about what it needs and when; perhaps juicy fruits or light smoothies in the morning, denser foods later, or sometimes simply water and rest.

If you're new to this journey, you may not notice these signals right away, and that's perfectly normal. Be patient. As your body lightens its toxic load and heals, the stronger "noise" of cravings or discomfort fades. With time, you'll start to hear the subtle, authentic messages of hunger, thirst, and balance that guide you toward true nourishment.

What Nutrition We Need

If I wanted to cover this topic fully, it could easily become a whole book on its own. I may write one in the future. For now, I'll give you a simple summary of the nutrition we need in our food. This is based on my experience and research and should be enough to guide your own exploration so you can find the optimal requirements for your personal needs and achieve the best possible level of health.

To thrive, we need **five main groups of nutrients**, along with **water** and **fibre**:

- **Water** is covered in a separate chapter.

- **Fibre**, though not broken down by the body, is essential for health. Think of it as a broom sweeping through your intestines, keeping things moving. On a natural lifestyle, you'll naturally get plenty of it.

Among the five groups, **three are macronutrients**; needed in large amounts daily:

1. Proteins

- **Role**: Build and repair tissues, muscles, enzymes, and hormones.

- **Natural sources**: Most fruits, Nuts (almonds, walnuts, Brazil nuts), seeds (chia, hemp, pumpkin, sunflower), leafy greens (Lettuce, spinach, kale), sprouts, and legumes (if tolerated).

2. Carbohydrates

- **Role**: Provide the body's main source of energy.

- **Natural sources**: Fruits (bananas, mangoes, dates, apples, grapes), starchy vegetables (carrots, beets), and leafy greens.

3. Lipids (Fats)

- **Role**: Essential for cell membranes, hormone balance, brain function, and absorption of fat-soluble vitamins (A, D, E, K).

- **Natural sources**: Seeds, avocados, coconuts, and nuts

The other **two are micronutrients**, required in smaller amounts but just as vital:

4. Vitamins

- **Role**: Act as catalysts for metabolism, immunity, and healthy cell reproduction.

- **Natural sources**:

    o   Vitamin C: citrus fruits, kiwis, berries.

    o   Vitamin A (as carotenoids): carrots, rockmelon, leafy greens.

    o   B vitamins: bananas, avocados, seeds, leafy greens.

    o   Vitamin K: kale, spinach, broccoli.

5. Minerals (Trace Elements)

- **Role**: Regulate electrolytes, enzyme function, oxygen transport, and countless other processes.

- **Natural sources**:

  o Zinc: pumpkin seeds, hemp seeds.

  o Iron: spinach, dried apricots, raisins.

  o Magnesium: leafy greens, almonds, chia seeds.

  o Calcium: figs, sesame seeds, kale, celery.

To function properly, we need carbohydrates for energy, and we need vitamins as catalysts to support metabolism, chemical reactions, and the reproduction of cells. We also need minerals such as zinc, iron, and copper for electrolyte balance, protein formation, and metabolic processes. In addition, amino acids and healthy fats (lipids) are required to build cells, proteins, muscle tissue, and enzymes. Some vitamins are fat-soluble, meaning they need fat to be absorbed effectively.

The good news is that you can get most of these nutrients from fresh and uncooked foods, primarily fruits, some vegetables, nuts, and seeds. Please note, I said most. Do you need supplements? In many cases, yes; but it depends on your body condition and where you live. Certain nutrients such as Vitamin B12, Vitamin D, and iodine are trickier, as they can be insufficient in almost any diet or lifestyle. Others, like omega-3 fatty acids, selenium, zinc, calcium, and iron, also require attention. These will be covered in more detail in the Supplement Chapter.

The reality is that our body is an incredible alchemist. Inside us is one of the most advanced chemical laboratories in the world, our liver. The liver is one of the body's most vital organs and acts as its central biochemical processing hub. It regulates metabolism, stores and releases energy, produces bile for fat digestion, and synthesises proteins essential for blood clotting and transport. Importantly, it also detoxifies harmful substances by breaking them down or converting them into forms that can be safely excreted. In this sense, the liver functions like the body's "chemical laboratory," constantly monitoring and adjusting thousands of reactions every day to keep us alive and in balance.

While the body can synthesise many substances it needs, an adequate intake of high-quality food remains essential. Interestingly, when I talk about this lifestyle, one of the first questions people often ask is: "How do you get your protein if you don't eat meat?"

Proteins

Well, It seems the meat industry with strong advertising support has done an excellent job of convincing people that protein is found only in meat. But think about it: when we eat beef, where did that cow get its protein? From meat? Of course not.

Yes, we need protein for cell repair and growth, but not nearly as much as is often advertised. Many TV ads and restaurant menus show oversized portions of steak or burgers, sometimes close to a kilogram per meal, suggesting this is the way to be "strong." What many don't realise is the strain such heavy meals can put on the digestive system.

Research suggests that adults need much less protein than commonly assumed; roughly 10–15% of daily calories to sustain cell reproduction and rebuild our muscles. Against the heavy advertisements, the main or only source of protein is not meat! Fruits, leafy veggies, nuts& seeds are excellent protein sources and they're often easier to digest than heavy meat meals.

Here's an important point: our bodies don't use "protein" directly. Instead, they break dietary proteins down into amino acids, and then rebuild them into the specific proteins our bodies need; whether that's for muscle, enzymes, hormones, or immune cells. In other words, we don't really need "protein from meat"; what we need are amino acids, which plants provide in abundance. Most proteins possess complex structures, with many still unknown to scientists. Additionally, there is ongoing research to uncover how our bodies create known proteins and clarify their various functions.

Some scientists argue that an optimal human diet must include meat due to its high protein content. They propose that human dietary habits have evolved over millions of years from primarily fruit consumption to the current ability to consume and digest a wide variety of foods available in the market. However, it's important to recognise that survival on a certain diet does not necessarily equate to optimal health. While humans may adapt to consuming alternative foods for survival, but adaptation doesn't automatically make a food ideal for long-term health.

Let's explore various diet categories, their distinctions, and which one is purportedly optimal for human health. Most mammals fall into four main categories: carnivores, omnivores, herbivores, and frugivores. The table in the next page is a brief comparison chart illustrating their differences, allowing you to determine which dietary pattern aligns best with human nature.

Table1: **Mammals Main Diets**

Diet	Carnivore	Omnivore	Herbivore	Frugivore	Human
Optimal Food	Meat	Meat and vegetable	Grass and tree foliage	Mainly fruits (may eat some vegetables &nuts)	**Your guess**
Mouth opening VS head size	Large	Large	Small	Small to Medium	Small
Jaw type	Lower Jaw embedded inside of upper jaw	Lower Jaw embedded inside of upper jaw	Upper jaw sits on the bottom jaw	Upper jaw sits on the bottom jaw	Upper jaw sits on the bottom jaw
Jaw Angle	Not expanded	Not expanded	Expanded	Expanded	Expanded
Necessity of chewing food	None; swallows food whole	Swallows food whole or simple crushing	Extensive chewing necessary	Chewing necessary	Chewing necessary
Facial muscles	Reduced to allow wide mouth gap	Reduced to allow wide mouth gap	Well-developed to facilitate chewing	Well-developed to facilitate chewing	Well-developed to facilitate chewing
Teeth (canines)	Long, sharp, and curved fangs	Long, sharp, and curved fangs	Rudimentary, dull, and short or none	Dull and short or long (for defense)	Rudimentary, short and blunted
Teeth (incisors)	Short and pointed	Short and pointed	Broad- Flattened and spade -shaped	Broad- Flattened and spade -shaped	Broad- Flattened and spade -shaped
Teeth(molars)	Sharp, jagged, and blade-shaped	Sharp blades and/or flattened	Flattened with cusps	Flattened with nodular cusps	Flattened with nodular cusps
Tongue	Extremely rough	Moderate to rough	Moderate to rough	Smooth	Smooth
Salivary gland size	Small	Small	Large	Large	Large
Salivary chemistry	Acidic	Acidic	Alkaline	Alkaline	Alkaline
Stomach acidity with food in it	pH around 1.5	pH around 1.5	pH 4 to 5	pH 4 to 5	pH 3.5 to 4.5
Stomach capacity	Over 60% of the total volume of digestive tract	Over 60% of the total volume of digestive tract	Less than 30% of the total volume of digestive tract	Less than 25% of the total volume of digestive tract	Less than 25% of the total volume of digestive tract
Peristalsis	Does not require fibre to stimulate	Does not require fibre to stimulate	Requires fibre to stimulate	Requires fibre to stimulate	Requires fibre to stimulate
Small intestine length	1.5 to 3 times body length	3 times body length	20 times body length	9 times body length	9 times body length
Colon length	Short	Short	Long	Long	Long
Colon chemistry	Alkaline	Alkaline	Acidic	Acidic	Acidic
Uricase enzyme	Secretion	Secretion	No secretion	No secretion	No secretion
Complete digestive time	2 to 4 hours	6 to 10 hours	24 to 48 hours	12 to 18 hours	12 to 18 hours
Circadian rhythm	Sleep 18-20 hours per day	Sleep 18-20 hours per day	Sleep less than 8 hours per day	Sleep 8 hours or less per day	Should sleep 8 hours or less per day
Nails	Sharp claws	Sharp claws or blunt hooves	Blunt hooves	Flattened nails	Flattened nails
Mammaries	Multiple teats	Multiple teats	Multiple teats	Dual breasts	Dual breasts

Sources: Various but mainly "Fruitarianism The Path to Paradise" Book by Anne Osborne and National Library of Medicine by USA Government.

As you can see in Table1, carnivores like lions, known for their meat-based diet, possess a relatively shorter small intestine, typically about a third of the length of a human's, ranging from 1 to 2.5 meters. Their digestive process is swift, with complete digestion occurring within 2 to 4 hours. In contrast, humans have a much longer small intestine, measuring approximately 5 to 7 meters, and our digestion takes considerably longer; in general, 12 to 18 hours, and sometimes more, depending on the food. Red meat, in particular, can take significantly longer for the body to fully process compared to fruits and vegetables. Meat contains complex protein molecules and breaking them down into amino acids requires more energy and time.

Unlike meat eaters, the human body lacks an enzyme called uricase, responsible for breaking down uric acid. Uricase breaks down uric acid into allantoin, a compound that is more easily excreted by the kidneys due to its high-water solubility. Without uricase, eating animal products can lead to excess uric acid, raising the risk of hyperuricemia. Hyperuricemia is a condition that can cause the formation of uric acid crystals, also known as urate crystals. These crystals have the potential to accumulate in the joints, causing gout, a painful type of arthritis. They can settle in the kidneys and contribute to the development of kidney stones.

If untreated, high uric acid levels may eventually lead to permanent bone, joint and tissue damage, kidney disease and heart disease. Research (see References) has also shown a link between high uric acid levels and type 2 diabetes, high blood pressure, and fatty liver disease.

Seafood and red meat are the main dietary sources of uric acid. Considering that we lack the enzyme to break them down efficiently, it's worth asking: are humans truly designed to be carnivore(meat eaters)?

I'm not sure what your guess is but based on my research and as you can explore Table1, I believe humans are not carnivore (meat eater) nor omnivores or herbivore, we are naturally frugivores. The type of our jaws, our stomach design, and the length and shape of our intestines are unlike any natural meat eater.

Humans evolved from the ape family, and in fact, the closest cousin we have in nature is a type of chimpanzee called the Bonobo, which has 98.8% of the same genes as human beings. You know what? Bonobo is a natural frugivore, which means they eat fruit as their primary food and some leaves and nuts as extra and main supplementation.

I couldn't find much study on their diet as, unfortunately, they are in danger of extinction, live in a remote area with dense jungles in Africa, and can only be reached by boats or push planes. Some research suggests they occasionally take animal products in small quantities, I imagine they should take them as supplements for some critical nutrition as they might not be available in their current fruit supplies.

Having discussed all the above, you can do your own research and explore whether the human body is truly designed to eat meat. The debate itself could fill an entire book, and that's not the purpose here. Many online resources and vegan scientists and doctors provide deeper insights into why reducing or avoiding meat may be beneficial.

While I acknowledge meat as a dense source of essential nutrients, as a quick thought experiment: if humans could naturally hunt an animal with bare hands, tear it apart, and genuinely enjoy eating every part raw; including the skin, flesh, bones, and organs perhaps then we could say we are natural carnivores. But in reality, our taste preferences and physiology suggest otherwise.

It's important to remember that humans likely turned to meat during times of necessity: the Ice Age, harsh climates, famine, or other survival pressures. Most studies (see References) indicate that early humans evolved in tropical Africa, an environment rich in wild fruit year-round, ideal for a frugivorous lifestyle. As groups migrated into deserts, colder regions, or less fertile areas, relying on animal foods may have been unavoidable.

Whatever the reasons, eating meat and animal products often creates digestive strain and increases the risk of chronic diseases. Our bodies can tolerate these foods for survival, but tolerance is not the same as thriving. Survival mode doesn't equal optimal health.

That's why I believe we should prioritise the foods nature clearly designed for us: fresh fruits, leafy greens, nuts, and seeds. If better and natural alternatives exist, why rely on foods that bring long-term risks?

And to be clear, this book is not mainly about arguing whether humans are "meat eaters" or "fruit eaters." My focus is on how nearly all our foods; whether meat, fruit, or vegetables are damaged when over-processed or oxidised by cooking. A simple rule of thumb: if you cannot eat a food in its natural state without fire, heavy processing, or artificial additions, maybe it's not meant to be your food.

Still, if someone chooses to eat meat, a gentler approach might be keeping it as close to its natural state as possible, raw or minimally processed, as seen in some cultures (e.g., sushi in Japan, or raw fish among the Inuit); or cooking it with lower temperatures; such as boiling or steaming (instead of frying and grilling). However, this still carries risks and consequences, and each person must weigh those for themselves.

Finally, always remember: cooking is burning, special at high temperature. Fire alters the structure of food, changing its chemistry and reducing its vitality. If left unchecked, fire consumes everything into ashes. That same principle applies to what we eat; the more we burn, the more we lose.

Now, let us go back to our protein discussion. Some studies (see References) suggest that, as adults, we only need around a maximum of 56 grams of combined amino acids per day, while other research indicates that less may be sufficient depending on individual needs. Our body needs 20 kinds of amino acids to create proteins. Nine of these are called "essential" because we must obtain them from food, while the body can synthesise the remaining eleven.

Most fruits contain essential amino acids. However, the quantities vary, and more research is needed to determine whether common fruits provide enough to meet daily needs. Some fruits, especially wild African fruits exceeding the RDI[1] of certain amino acids. For example, jacket plum has unusually high lysine content, and a study by the University of Johannesburg found that Halleria lucida contained particularly high amounts of isoleucine, leucine, phenylalanine, and valine; in some cases exceeding WHO[2] Guidelines.

Bananas, well known for containing tryptophan (an essential amino acid), provide only 7 of the 9 essential amino acids and are particularly low in isoleucine and methionine. My understanding is although some of the fruits have a good content of amino acids in general, they are poor enough to supply all recommended daily

---

[1] Recommended Daily Intake usually set by the World Health Organisation

[2] World Health Organisation

intake of the essential ones unless you eat a high volume of them, which is not practical, for example, 50 bananas a day!

I believe we need to eat a small quantity of seeds, nuts, and some vegetables to ensure adequate intake of all amino acids. Part of the challenge is that modern industrial agriculture depletes soil quality, so today's fruits and vegetables may not contain the same nutrient density as wild foods available to our ancestors.

Chia seed has all nine essential amino acids and eight non-essential ones. Hemp seeds have all 20 amino acids in reasonable quantity; both are called complete proteins. Interestingly, hemp seed has a higher rate of 32 g of protein per 100 g, while red meat is about 26 g per 100 g. Dried spirulina powder which is type of algae can supply about 60 grams of protein per 100 grams. Yet, when most people think of protein, they think of butchers rather than plant-based sources.

Both chia and hemp seeds are great for optimal health; the best protein sources and a combination of both will give us the required fatty acids, which will be discussed in the lipid section.

Grains such as soy, quinoa, and buckwheat each contain all nine essential amino acids, making them a complete source of amino acids for our body to make its required proteins. Quinoa, in addition, contains 7 out of 11 of the non-essential amino acids, which makes it a superfood for body protein needs.

However, I do not personally recommend frequent consumption of grains. While their sprouts are accepted by many Raw Vegan practitioners, grains can be hard to digest and may contribute to other issues. Plants often protect their seeds with "anti-nutrients" (like phytates and lectins), which can reduce mineral absorption and enzyme function. Germination (sprouting) can reduce some of these compounds, but they are still not as easy to digest as fruits, vegetables, nuts, or seeds.

I prefer sprouted legumes such as lentils, chickpeas, and mung beans. Sprouted quinoa, though technically a pseudo grain, behaves more like a legume in terms of nutrition and makes an excellent addition to the diet. These sprouts not only provide a broad spectrum of amino acids but also supply essential trace elements that support overall health.

Walnuts, almonds, hazelnuts, and pistachios all contain the nine essential amino acids, and in general, 2 cups of combination of these four nuts supply all the essential amino acids we need. Brazil nuts are also a good company with the above four nuts, which contain a good quantity of methionine, an essential amino acid, which is less in the other nuts. But nuts also need to be eaten moderately for two reasons: firstly, they contain fats (especially Omega-6 and Omega-9), and secondly, they are hard to digest. They usually cause problems in the body if consumed in large amounts. If it is decided to be consumed, both nuts and seeds must be in a Raw and natural state.

It is recommended to soak them for at least 24 hours to activate them, making them more bioavailable and accessible for digestion.

I hope I have given several fruit and plant alternatives to the meat, which can provide us with enough amino acids. There are many vegan athletes and special bodybuilders, which you can find by searching online and checking how they build their muscles from plants. Even most of the other body builders who eat meat use protein powders to build their muscles. Do you think those powders are all made from animal products? From what I know many are made from plants!

As another piece of evidence, consider the animals with the highest muscle mass on our planet and whether they are carnivores or herbivores. For example, compare a lion to an elephant. How many muscles does an elephant have, and what kind of food fuels their development? Now, consider a gorilla. How much muscle mass does a gorilla possess, and how strong is this animal? It's worth noting how easily a gorilla can break a coconut with its hands. I believe any creature on Earth, if it adheres to the diet nature designed for it, will be in its strongest condition within the limits of its genetic makeup. Conversely, consuming the undesired foods can weaken the body and diminish its strength.

I hope this clears up one of the most common questions: *"Where does a Raw Vegan diet get its protein?"* The truth is, plants provide all the amino acids we need; just as they do for the strongest animals on Earth. Protein should never be your biggest worry when eating a natural, balanced diet. Focus instead on fresh, living foods, and protein will take care of itself.

Now, let's look at another nutrient that causes just as much confusion, carbohydrates.

Carbohydrates

Carbohydrates (commonly called carbs) are another controversial macronutrient. There's been a lot of debate in the health community about whether we actually *need* carbs or whether we should cut them out completely. The low-carb, no-carb, or keto[1] diet? You've probably heard of them, and maybe felt just as confused as I once did. This confusion usually comes from the link between carbs, sugar, and conditions like diabetes.

Excessive and processed carbs are often stored in the body as fat, which is why many people with raised bellies worry that eating

---

[1] Keto is a diet high in fat and low carb, which forces the body to burn fat.

more carbs will only make things worse. But let's dig deeper and see what our bodies really need.

As you might have guessed, carbohydrates are molecules made from carbon, hydrogen, and oxygen atoms. They are primarily sugars and starches, and are found in nearly every food group except *meat* and *eggs*. (A handy talking point for animal-product advocates who like to scare people away from carbs, isn't it?)

Carbohydrates are generally classified according to how quickly they are digested and absorbed in the body. The two main categories are:

- **Simple carbohydrates** — commonly found in biscuits, cookies, chocolates, and packaged fruit juices. They contain simple sugars like fructose, galactose, and glucose, but usually **lack fibre.** They digest quickly, causing a rapid spike in blood sugar followed by a sharp crash. These sugars are often heated, processed, and degraded, which is why they can cause a range of physical and psychological problems when eaten regularly. Some research (see References) even suggests that they provide an easy source of fuel for unhealthy cells, including cancer cells.

- **Complex carbohydrates (polysaccharides)** — made up of two or more simple sugars linked together. They take longer to break down, releasing energy more steadily. Complex carbs are found in grains, legumes, nuts, vegetables, and fruits like bananas, berries, and apples.

Glucose, a simple sugar, is the body's primary source of energy for the brain and central nervous system. If carbohydrates are eliminated from the diet, as some people attempt, the body must work harder to create glucose from other nutrients (through processes like gluconeogenesis). This puts extra strain on the liver and digestive organs.

The importance of glucose as an energy source cannot be overstated. It is vital not only for the brain and nervous system but also for the kidneys, red blood cells, and muscles. Even while we sleep, the body relies on glucose to regulate body temperature, support digestion, and keep the heart beating. Unlike some other sugars, natural glucose is readily broken down and absorbed, providing clean energy with minimal stress on the system.

In contrast, **processed and damaged carbohydrates** like white bread, cooked rice, or burnt potatoes (e.g., French fries) deliver little nutritional value. Worse, they can generate harmful byproducts such as **acrylamide,** which stresses body cells.

Highly processed sweets such as chocolates, biscuits, cookies, lollies, and pre-made packaged foods; go even further. They not only contain refined sugars but are often loaded with artificial colours, preservatives, and chemical additives.

It's interesting how often products loaded with refined sugars show up in daily life. Even highly educated human including doctors and scientists; may consume them regularly. In fact, it's not unusual to see bowls of sweets or candies in medical offices, which highlights just how deeply processed sugars are woven into modern culture.

Processed sugars, produced through heating and crystallisation in industrial sugar mills, place extra strain on the body and can be difficult to digest. Over time, they may contribute to cellular stress and are considered by many researchers to have toxic effects when consumed regularly. Whether labelled white, brown, raw, or cane, the difference is minimal; all involve extraction and heating that alter their natural state.

Although some forms are marketed as "healthier," once sugar is removed from its original source and refined through heat, it loses much of its natural balance. As discussed throughout this book, fire and high-heat processing change food at a structural level; a change that ultimately works against long-term health.

Returning to our initial point, whole fruits are one of the best natural sources of carbohydrates. With their natural sugars and fibre, they provide steady fuel for our organs; especially the brain and nervous system; while supporting the smooth function of other body systems. This type of fuel is easily burned and converted into energy, without overburdening the body.

Glucose is the body's primary source of fuel. Once carbohydrates are digested, glucose enters the bloodstream, and the pancreas releases insulin to help cells absorb it. Beyond the brain and nerves, muscles, kidneys, and even the eyes rely on glucose for energy.

Glucose metabolism is carefully regulated, with the liver playing a central role in balancing blood sugar. Hormones like leptin also signal satiety, usually about 20 minutes after eating; one reason why eating slowly can help prevent overeating. The body stores excess glucose as glycogen in the liver and muscles, which can be drawn upon during fasting or exercise. Once glycogen stores are full, surplus glucose is converted into fat.

When this balance tips too far, problems arise: prolonged high blood sugar can damage blood vessels and organs, while very low levels can cause dizziness, fatigue, or even seizures. To counter dips, hormones like glucagon and adrenaline trigger the liver to release glucose and preserve supply for the brain.

So, should we fear carbohydrates? The answer is no; but we should respect the *type* of carbohydrates we consume. Fruits are an excellent choice: they contain natural sugars, fibre that slows absorption, and a wide range of vitamins and minerals. Eating fruits with their skins where appropriate (like pears, apples, and peaches) adds even more fibre and nutrients.

Personally, I'm not a fan of fruit juices because juicing strips away fibre. Smoothies are a better option if you prefer a processed version, as they retain the fibre. Still, it's best to keep in mind that processing accelerates oxidation; and the closer food is to its natural state, the better for your health.

There are some talks in the medical industry that fruit sugar harms the body and that fruit consumption should be minimised to avoid diabetes. I've even seen people told to avoid carbs altogether and eat mostly protein instead. Some health professionals believe low- or no-carb diets are the best way to control blood sugar. From my understanding, this isn't correct. Many parts of our body; especially the brain; can only use glucose as their fuel.

Even if we consume only protein, the liver must convert it into glucose for vital organs to function. This does not solve the problem; it simply shifts the burden to the digestive system, which must work harder to break down complex protein molecules. By contrast, natural fruit sugars are easily digested and require little processing.

The real issue lies in the gradual decline of pancreatic beta cell function; a fact often overlooked when the focus is placed only on carb-counting and blood sugar spikes. High levels of fat in the blood also reduce the ability of cells to absorb glucose, which is another major factor in diabetes.

You may find it surprising that even refined sugars don't usually harm cells directly. Instead, they react with fats and proteins to form harmful compounds such as Advanced Glycation End Products (AGEs) and Glycated LDL (GLDL). These compounds can damage pancreatic beta cells, accelerating the onset of diabetes.

By the time most people are diagnosed with diabetes, 70–80% of their beta cells may already be lost. As I've discussed earlier in this book, glands are among the first parts of the body affected by toxins from unhealthy foods. Beta cells are particularly vulnerable because they have relatively low antioxidant defences compared to other cell types. This makes them more sensitive to oxidative stress, especially from oxidised and processed foods and the free radicals they create.

Whole fruits, rich in antioxidants, help defend beta cells against this stress. Research (see References) has shown that eating whole fruits can lower the risk of Type 2 diabetes, and I have personally seen people improve their condition; even heal by following a natural lifestyle and removing the unhealthy foods from their plates.

I hope I could answer one of the main questions people with diabetes often have about fruit sugar. However, if you are starting a natural lifestyle journey and already have diabetes, it is **wise** to focus on fruits with more fibre and less sugar. Also add more leafy greens, to help reduce blood sugar spikes. This can support your body until the pancreas has a chance to heal and beta cell function improves, allowing for more stable insulin production.

People sometimes ask me whether potatoes or rice are necessary as sources of carbohydrates in a Raw diet. My response is usually simple:

"Do we really need to eat everything? Why do humans think they must consume every single food or creature on Earth? Shouldn't we consider that, like all animals, we are also part of nature; and nature has already designed the right foods for us?"

I once heard someone joke that humans can eat everything that flies except aeroplanes, and everything in the ocean except submarines. Funny, but should we really take that as advice?

Even within a Raw Vegan community, it isn't necessary to consume every single item growing in a garden. What essential nutrient is in potatoes that isn't already found in fruits or vegetables? Or what unique compound does eggplant offer that you cannot get elsewhere?

And sometimes some people ask about potato chips! And how they can ignore this delicious treat if they become Raw Vegan!

Well, I suggest they do their own research and find out what is inside potato chips. Can they find anything healthy in it? I am sure you can find the three most significant types of unhealthy ingredients in it:

1. Highly oxidised carbs,
2. Highly heated and full complex of damaged oil,
3. And high salt level

The last one is interesting, as always it is. Do the test tonight and make your favourite potato chips. Do not add any salt and see how delicious it will be. I love to hear about your experience!

Same thing for rice and bread. The only difference can be the heat intensity, leading to less food damage and reduced chance of harm to your body.

To wrap up this chapter, let me be clear: carbohydrates are the last thing you should worry about when following a natural lifestyle. The only concern arises if you're not eating enough fresh, raw fruit each day. When your plate is full of colourful, fresh, raw foods, carbohydrates stop being a problem and become pure fuel for energy, clarity, and life itself.

Lipids or Fats

Fat, what a topic! Is it good or bad for our health? What comes to mind when you hear the word "fat"? Maybe someone overweight with a raised tummy, or a greasy steak dripping into a fire? Or perhaps the satisfaction of spreading a rich, fatty butter over toast followed by the guilt after a heavy, greasy meal like a burger.

Whatever your feeling, fats; or lipids play essential roles in our body. Like carbs, some people think we should delete fats from our lives to stay healthy. That's a misconception.

While you might have heard people are dying from conditions associated with obesity and extra body fat, fat is one of the macronutrients essential for our body functions.

Fat is present in every single cell of our body; without it, we wouldn't survive. The membrane of all our cells is made of fat; nearly 60 per cent of our brain is fat, and fat in the form of cholesterol (lipoprotein) protects our neurons and our nervous system. And yet, *cholesterol* is such a scary word you hear almost every day from doctors, magazines, and the news!

Fat has eight main essential functions in the body:

- Regulating body temperature
- Energy storage (excess carbs converted into fat in body adipose tissue and later can be used as fuel when needed)
- Supporting bone health
- Critical for brain cells
- Absorption of fat-soluble Vitamins A, D, E & K
- Insulation of cells
- Protection of internal organs such as the heart and kidneys by making a cushion around them

- Essential for hormone production such as leptin

Chemically, fats are made of hydrogen, carbon, oxygen, and a small compound called glycerol. The main dietary fats are:

- **Triglycerides** (over 90% of dietary fat)

- **Phospholipids**

- **Sterols** (cholesterol, phytosterols, etc.)

Triglycerides are further divided:

- **Saturated fats** → mostly from animal products, some plants like coconut oil. Solid at room temp.

- **Unsaturated fats** → usually from plants, liquid at room temp (e.g., olive oil).

  - **Monounsaturated (Omega-9)** → body can make these, so not "essential."

  - **Polyunsaturated (Omega-3 & Omega-6)** → *essential* because the body cannot make them.

Trans fats primarily come from animal products like dairy and meat, though in smaller amounts. Artificial trans fatty acids are predominantly found in plant source oils that have been partially hydrogenated. Also **overheated oils** (frying, baking at high temps, especially re-used oils) can generate trans fats and other harmful oxidation products. Both natural and artificial trans fatty acids are considered harmful and should be minimised or eliminated from the diet and lifestyle.

Monounsaturated fatty acids are often referred to as Omega-9 fatty acids, but they are non-essential because the body can synthesise them from other fats.

Polyunsaturated fatty acids are categorised into two:

- **Omega-6**: widely available in both plant oils and animal products. Usually over-consumed in the modern diet.
- **Omega-3**: far less common, but critical. Anti-inflammatory, supports heart, brain, and immune health.

These two **cannot be synthesised** in the body and must be taken from our food.

Some animal fats and plant oils are good sources of Omega-6 fatty acids, and there are few concerns about them.

However, Omega-3 is the tricky one as the source of it is limited to some seafood and some plants. Given the confusion surrounding the importance of fats for our health, let's recap our discussion. While there's a lot to understand about fats and fatty acids, for practical purposes, the key takeaway is to focus on Omega-3 and Omega-6 fatty acids. Omega-6 is generally abundant in most diets and lifestyle choices, so it's less of a concern. However, Omega-3 is crucial and requires attention. Ensuring an adequate intake of Omega-3 fatty acids is important for overall health.

Most research (see References) suggests that achieving a balanced ratio of Omega-6 to Omega-3 fatty acids, ideally around 1:1[1], is important for optimal health.

However in many modern diets, the ratio is imbalanced, with Omega-6 intake typically exceeding Omega-3 intake. This imbalance can lead to chronic inflammation in the body, as Omega-6 fatty acids are pro-inflammatory when consumed in excess.

---

[1] There are some sources advise that the ratio of 4:1 of Omega-6 to Omega-3 is still healthy.

Research (see References) shows that in some individuals, Omega-6 intake can be up to 17 times higher than Omega-3 intake, further worsening the imbalance.

While olive oil is often regarded as one of the healthiest oils, it contains little to no Omega-3 fatty acids. Despite its many benefits and the widespread recommendations by scientists and health professionals, olive oil should not be considered a source of essential Omega-3.

Omega-6 fatty acids, on the other hand, are important for certain bodily functions, particularly in regulating inflammation. However, when consumed in excess, they can tip the balance and contribute to chronic inflammation.

Conversely, Omega-3 fatty acids are valued for their anti-inflammatory properties. While fruits like avocado contain mainly Omega-6 and Omega-9 fatty acids, only a few fruits; such as guava and papaya, provide trace amounts of Omega-3 (ALA). However, these levels are far too low to meet daily requirements, which is why nuts, seeds, and algae are the key plant-based sources.

Omega-3 fatty acids consist of three main types all of which are essential for various bodily functions:

- **Alpha-Linolenic Acid (ALA),**
- **Eicosapentaenoic Acid (EPA)**
- **Docosahexaenoic Acid (DHA)**

Alpha-Linolenic Acid (ALA) is primarily found in fruits and plants, while Eicosapentaenoic Acid (EPA) and Docosahexaenoic Acid (DHA) are commonly sourced from seaweed, algae and fish.

Although our bodies can convert ALA into EPA and DHA, this conversion process is inefficient; typically less than 10% for EPA and under 5% for DHA. Factors such as age, sex, genetics, and especially a high intake of Omega-6 can make this conversion even less effective. Because of this, a higher intake of ALA (around 2,000–3,000 mg daily) is often recommended to support adequate EPA and DHA levels.

Microalgae (the original source of EPA and DHA for fish) can provide these fatty acids directly. While foods like seaweed, nori, spirulina, and chlorella offer valuable nutrients, only certain algae-based oils reliably supply meaningful amounts of EPA and DHA.

Among raw plant sources, chia seeds, flaxseeds, and hemp seeds are the richest in ALA. Just two tablespoons of chia seeds plus two tablespoons of hemp seeds can supply enough Omega-3 to balance with Omega-6 intake. Adding small amounts of walnuts or other nuts can also contribute, but moderation is key to avoid tipping the ratio toward Omega-6.

Creamy tropical fruits, seeds, and nuts can help support essential fatty acid intake, but for many people; especially those on long-term raw vegan diets; a high-quality algae-based DHA/EPA supplement may still be the best way to ensure optimal levels.

Vitamins

Vitamins are certainly a fascinating topic, aren't they? There's endless discussion about their importance, and it sometimes feels as though people take comfort in swallowing several multivitamin supplements each day; even though we also hear warnings about the risks of excessive intake. Let's take a closer look at this remarkable subject.

The word *vitamin* comes from the Latin *vita*, meaning *life*. These are essential micronutrients that our bodies need in small amounts to function properly. There are 13 recognised essential vitamins: **A, the B group, C, D, E, and K.** They are involved in everything from metabolism and hormone regulation to cell reproduction, bone and tissue maintenance, and detoxification. Some vitamins must be obtained daily because the body doesn't store them, while others can be stored for longer periods.

Vitamins do not directly provide energy, but they act as catalysts and coenzymes in countless metabolic processes. They support the breakdown of carbohydrates, fats, and proteins, and many serve as antioxidants, helping to neutralise harmful oxidative by-products. This is one reason why people with T.W.D. and high in processed foods, are often encouraged to increase their vitamin intake to help counter oxidative stress and free radicals.

Vitamins fall into two broad groups: **water-soluble** and **fat-soluble.** Water-soluble vitamins (like vitamin C and the B group) dissolve in water and are not stored in large amounts in the body. Fat-soluble vitamins (A, D, E, and K) need fat for absorption and can be stored in fatty tissue or the liver. Importantly, vitamins and minerals often work in synergy. For example:

- Vitamin C enhances iron absorption.

- Vitamins A and E function more effectively together.

- Folate (B9) works best when zinc is also present.

This principle of **nutrient synergy** means that a varied, balanced diet is far more effective than relying on isolated supplements.

At the same time, certain nutrients can compete for absorption. For instance, zinc and copper use the same transport pathways in the gut, meaning too much zinc can block copper absorption. Similarly, very high doses of vitamin C may interfere with vitamin

B12 stability. This is one reason why "all-in-one" tablets claiming to provide most or all vitamins and minerals are not always ideal.

A healthy, natural diet of unprocessed fruits and vegetables should be the foundation, with supplements used only to cover specific gaps.

Water-soluble vitamins are particularly fragile: they break down easily in the presence of **oxygen, light,** and **especially heat.** That's why prolonged cooking or storage can destroy much of their value. For example, vitamin C is highly unstable and degrades quickly when exposed to heat or air. This sensitivity connects with what we've already discussed; heating food often damages its nutrients, sometimes even turning antioxidants into harmful pro-oxidants.

Due to time constraints, many people opt for pre-cut fruits or packaged juices, believing them to be healthy choices. However, studies show that once fruit is cut, vitamin C begins to degrade rapidly; for example, a single cut in an orange may reduce its vitamin C content by up to 15%. Similarly, a head of broccoli can lose more than half of its vitamin C after just a few days of storage or transport. Now imagine what happens to pre-cut fruit packs sitting on supermarket shelves.

Cooking fruit accelerates this process even further. Making jams or compotes destroys much of their vitamin C and other heat-sensitive nutrients. It's surprising that some health textbooks still label "no-added-sugar jams" as a healthy option simply because of the natural fruit sugars.

Water-soluble vitamins like vitamin C and most of the B group are abundant in fresh fruits and leafy greens. However, vitamin B12 is an exception and remains a challenge, which I'll discuss later in the supplement chapter.

Fat-soluble vitamins (A, D, E, and K) require fat for proper absorption. They are usually carried in the bloodstream by protein transporters and, if taken in excess, can be stored in the liver or fatty tissues. Unlike water-soluble vitamins, they are not quickly excreted through the kidneys, which means excess supplementation can sometimes lead to toxicity, especially affecting the liver. These vitamins are more heat-resistant than water-soluble ones, but they are still best preserved in their natural, unheated form.

One important exception is vitamin D, which we cannot reliably obtain from plant foods alone. Sunlight exposure remains the primary natural source of vitamin D, and I'll explain more in the supplement chapter.

I won't go into detailed functions or Recommended Daily Intake (RDI) here, as that would be another book in itself. The key is this: a varied diet of fresh, unprocessed fruits and vegetables should be your foundation, with supplements used only to cover specific gaps. Reliable resources; and my own website articles can guide you further on your journey.

Please note: the RDI (Recommended Daily Intake) is designed as a general guide for the average population, most of whom follow the Typical Western Diet (T.W.D.). While it is a helpful benchmark, it may not always reflect the needs of individuals following a natural or raw lifestyle. Depending on your condition, age, location, and the availability of fresh fruits and vegetables, you may require more(or sometimes less) than the standard recommendation.

The same is true for blood test "reference ranges." These ranges are built statistically from large groups of people eating conventional diets, and they serve as averages rather than personalised targets. For example, many raw vegans show slightly lower blood iron levels compared with standard references, yet remain perfectly healthy if other markers like haemoglobin and energy levels are stable. Similarly, Vitamin D can show up slightly higher in individuals with proper sun exposure, which is expected and not necessarily a problem.

In short, RDIs and blood test ranges are useful tools but not absolute rules. They give a baseline for the general public, but your personal results should be interpreted in the context of your lifestyle, diet, and overall health. That's why it's best to monitor trends over time and, where needed, discuss them with a trusted health professional who understands nutrition beyond the standard T.W.D. framework.

Minerals

Minerals can be found everywhere, from the table salt people use every day or in mining operations where valuable minerals are extracted from the Earth's depths for use in a wide range of products and structures. From a health perspective, our bodies require minerals in small daily doses, some of which are smaller than the head of a pin.

Despite their tiny size, these minerals are vital for our well-being, crucial for the optimal functioning of our cells. They play essential roles, from maintaining electrolyte balance to supporting bone formation. You're probably familiar with major minerals like calcium, iron, and sodium. Minerals have two categories: major (or macrominerals) and trace elements (or microminerals).

The known macro-minerals that the body needs more than 100 mg or more each day are:

- Calcium
- Magnesium
- Sulphur
- Potassium
- Sodium
- Phosphorus
- Chloride

The microminerals or trace elements we need less than 100 mg each day are:

- Iron
- Zinc
- Selenium
- Chromium
- Manganese
- Fluoride
- Iodine
- Copper
- Boron
- Molybdenum

You may recall seeing bottles labeled as electrolytes or others marketed for bone and teeth health in supermarkets; these products highlight the primary functions of minerals in the body. Essential electrolytes in the body serve several critical functions, including maintaining pH (see Glossary) balance, which is vital for overall health, regulating body fluids such as lymph and blood, and facilitating the transmission of messages between cells through their electric charges.

The main electrolytes are made from calcium, magnesium, chloride, sodium, and potassium dissolved in water. As mentioned, they prepare either positive or negative ions for their bodily functions. Other than these, minerals are essential in building and maintaining cells. You might have heard that calcium is the main mineral required for bones and teeth, with the help of Vitamin D, proteins, phosphorus, and fluoride.

Many minerals function most effectively when accompanied by specific vitamins, and at times, they may compete with each other for absorption if consumed simultaneously and in unbalanced quantities.

For those following T.W.D. the body often becomes more **acidic** due to frequent intake of animal products and low-pH foods like meat, dairy, sodas, coffee, and tea. To buffer this acidity, the body may draw on calcium reserves from the bones, contributing to conditions like osteoporosis[1]. This helps explain why such bone diseases are more common in countries with high dairy and meat consumption, such as the USA and Australia.

Returning to our discussion, I won't dive into the full details of minerals, their functions, or all the ways to get them naturally; that could easily fill another book of its own. I encourage you to do your own research, and I'll also share more information on my website for those who want to explore further.

The good news is that with a natural lifestyle, a healthy body, and a strong gut, you'll meet most of your mineral needs from fresh fruits, vegetables, nuts, and seeds. Still, there are exceptions. Some trace elements are less abundant in modern soils; especially in heavily farmed areas, and may require extra attention through supplementation. Being mindful of this helps ensure your body stays in balance.

---

[1] Osteoporosis is a disease in which the body loses bone mass, and it usually affects people aged over 50. (See Glossary)

The Overlooked Nutrients

While the classic essential nutrients: carbohydrates, proteins, fats, vitamins, minerals, (plus water and fibre) cover the bulk of what the body needs, there are other lesser-known compounds that are just as vital for specific functions.

These are often referred to as "conditionally essential" nutrients as our body can usually produce them, but not always in sufficient quantities, especially in times of stress, ageing, illness, or sometimes in a raw vegan lifestyle.

Let's look at some of the most important ones:

Choline which is formally acknowledged in 1998 is sometimes grouped with B vitamins, but it plays distinct roles in:

- Brain development and memory

- Formation of cell membranes

- Liver function and fat metabolism

- Production of acetylcholine, a neurotransmitter for muscle control and cognition

Choline deficiency can lead to memory issues, muscle damage, and fatty liver.

Brussels sprouts, broccoli, cauliflower, sunflower seeds, and quinoa are good sources of choline. In particular, sunflower lecithin is an excellent source that fits well within a raw vegan diet.

Carnitine (L-carnitine) Carnitine's primary role is transporting fatty acids into mitochondria, where they're burned for energy.

Although the body can synthesise it, infants, older adults, and people under stress may not make enough.

Plant-based diets can support its production when rich in B vitamins and amino acids.

Coenzyme Q10 (CoQ10) a powerful antioxidant which is involved in cellular energy production, particularly within the mitochondria.

While not officially essential, CoQ10 levels decline with age and in people with chronic diseases, making it functionally essential for heart and brain health.

Taurine supports neurological development, eye health, and fluid balance.

It's not found in plant foods, but most healthy individuals can synthesise it from sulfur-containing amino acids. Still, it's worth noting for those on long-term vegan or raw diets.

Inositol (formerly called vitamin B8) Involved in cell signalling, insulin sensitivity, and mood regulation.

It's naturally found in fruits, beans, and whole grains, and is sometimes used therapeutically for PCOS and anxiety.

Alpha-Lipoic Acid (ALA) is a unique antioxidant that helps regenerate other antioxidants (like vitamin C and E) and plays a role in energy metabolism.

The body produces it in small amounts, but demand may increase with age or illness. Found in vegetables like spinach and broccoli.

Other Vitamin-like Compounds includes PABA, biopterin, carnosine, and others. They support enzyme function, tissue repair, and metabolic balance, but are not always classified as essential because the body typically produces them unless under stress or genetic limitation.

How to Eat

So far, we've explored why we eat, when to eat, and what nutrition our bodies need. But there's another key factor: **how we eat.** The way we approach food directly affects nutrient absorption and even how much we enjoy it.

Have you noticed your mouth watering at the sight (or even thought) of your favourite food? That's your brain priming the digestive system for action.

The first thing we should all remember is that our stomachs do not have teeth, right? The only place in our body equipped with teeth is the mouth. Their role goes far beyond creating a pleasant smile. Teeth are precision tools designed to bite, grind, and break down food into smaller pieces, making it easier to mix with saliva and prepare for digestion.

When food is chewed thoroughly, it becomes liquified and infused with saliva before being swallowed. This step is not optional; it's the foundation of proper digestion. Saliva doesn't just moisten food; it contains powerful enzymes. The most important is **amylase**, which starts breaking down carbohydrates into simple sugars, and **lingual lipase**, which begins the process of fat digestion. By chewing properly, you give these enzymes time to act, transforming food into a form your stomach can handle.

On the other hand, chewing your food properly allows your stomach enough time to release gastric juices for thorough digestion. The brain recognises the type of food through signals from the mouth and sends instructions to the digestive organs to prepare the appropriate juices, determine their intensity, and produce the specific enzymes required for proper digestion.

Ghrelin, a stomach hormone, signals hunger to the brain, prompting us to eat. In addition, another hormone produced in the stomach after we eat, called leptin, communicates satiety with the brain. It is said that 20 minutes of eating is when leptin signals the brain to stop eating.

Chewing well and eating slowly will give the body enough time to respond and manage the eating properly.

Now you understand how important it is to eat our food slowly by chewing it thoroughly and breaking it down properly.

You might have seen people rushing around with fast foods, trying to save time, but they may not realise how fast eating can strain digestion and contribute to post-meal bloating. Fast eating also often leads to overeating, as leptin signalling doesn't have enough time to register. When this becomes a habit, the brain begins to ignore leptin's signal altogether, and food intake can easily surpass the body's actual needs.

The other benefit of slow eating is the joy and pleasure it brings. As mentioned before, when you align with a natural lifestyle and consume food that meets your body's pure cellular needs, your senses become sharper. One of our most treasured senses is taste. By eating slowly and chewing thoroughly, you can fully appreciate the flavours of clean, raw, and mostly unprocessed meals which not only provide energy but also genuine satisfaction.

Eating with patience, chewing thoroughly, and keeping a relaxed mind; ideally in a quiet space with minimal talk or distractions is the key to optimal absorption and digestion. Follow this simple habit whenever possible, and you'll find meals more nourishing and enjoyable.

Drinking Water

In addition to all the above, our body requires another essential substance, water, for its activities and survival. Many market products claim to be human drinks, along with countless articles about water's ideal consumption for maximum benefits, leading to confusion. I will try my best to make it simple for you from my understanding.

The first and most important fact is that our bodies need water; humans generally cannot survive longer than seven days without it. Approximately 60–70% of our body mass is water, filling all our tissues and organs. We require this vital substance for all our physical activities and receive thirst signals when it is needed. Water plays a crucial role in blood and lymph circulation, as well as in maintaining the body's electrolyte balance.

Not drinking enough water can lead to dehydration, which can be identified by the colour of urine. Normally, urine should be a pale-yellow colour; if it appears darker yellow, it may indicate dehydration, while very clear urine may suggest overhydration. One exception is during extensive detoxification (detox), when urine may become darker as the body eliminates toxins.

Our body uses water for almost every function, and a lack of it can lead to life-threatening situations, such as kidney failure or heat stroke. Another crucial role of water is supporting detoxification, helping organs filter and eliminate waste products.

Excessive water consumption can also be dangerous, potentially leading to a life-threatening condition known as hyponatremia. This sometimes occurs in athletes who drink excessively to stay ahead of thirst. Our bodies need to maintain a balance of minerals, such as sodium and potassium, known as electrolytes, which are essential for proper function. Excess water can dilute these electrolytes, particularly sodium, which is vital for the nervous system. To minimise the risk of health issues, drinking an appropriate amount of water regularly when thirsty is better than consuming very large amounts at once.

The amount of water we need daily differs from person to person, considering the environment in which they live, the temperature and humidity of the air, their age, food intake, activities, etc. You might have heard an adult requires eight glasses of water daily, which equals around 2 litres. It's beneficial for some, but not all.

People following a T.W.D. may require more water than those who adhere to a natural lifestyle. This is because the body of individuals on the T.W.D. needs extra fluid to help dilute and eliminate the higher load of waste products. A minimum of 8 glasses or more of water may be the correct recommendation for someone on such a diet, especially if it includes a lot of heat-damaged and processed food. However, individuals with a natural lifestyle should rely more on interpreting their body's natural thirst signals.

Many people also drink while eating. From my understanding, this is one of the least helpful drinking habits someone can develop. Almost all eateries serve food with drinks, and it's common to see people having a hot burger with a cold Coke in their hands; eating and drinking together. This widespread practice, particularly among those who eat mostly processed foods, can interfere with digestion and may even worsen issues such as constipation.

I used to have the same habit when I was younger and followed what was considered a standard diet. I recall experiencing stomach pain after each meal, which I assumed was natural. From an engineering mindset, I thought a working process required some pressure; and to me, stomach pressure meant pain! At times, the pain was so intense that I had to take painkillers to alleviate it. Have you ever experienced something similar?

Let's look more closely at the effects of drinking while eating. When food enters the stomach, it needs to be broken down by stomach acid and enzymes so it can be prepared for absorption in the intestines. This process actually begins before the first bite, as soon as we see food on the table or smell it, with the body priming itself for digestion.

When we drink water during meals, stomach acid can be diluted, which may reduce its effectiveness in breaking down food. Poorly digested food leads to two main issues:

1. **Slower processing** – Food may remain in the intestines longer, increasing the chance of constipation. Constipation itself is not just uncomfortable but also creates an environment where harmful bacteria can thrive.

2. **Reduced nutrient absorption** – If food isn't properly digested, the body cannot extract enough nutrients, leaving much of the nutrition unused. This weakens the body's defence systems and can make us more vulnerable to illness.

As a simple demonstration, if you are on a T.W.D., try this test: take a piece of cooked, greasy food like a barbecued steak or burger, pour a cold Coke over it, and watch. I did this years ago and saw the meat turn rubbery. Now, imagine your stomach trying to process something that behaves like rubber inside you!

This is why some health practitioners recommend spacing out drinks, at least half an hour before and about two hours after meals; especially for those on the T.W.D. I would also suggest this practice for people following a natural lifestyle, with some adjustments outlined below.

The first thing to note is that the best drink for humans is pure water. Not every beverage sold in supermarkets qualifies as a "drink" for the human body, as many contain chemical additives. In my view, the purest water comes directly from fruit. I'm not suggesting fruit juice, but rather whole fruits. When you eat fruit, you may find you hardly need to drink additional water; depending on the fruit's water content, the season, temperature, and your activity level. The water inside high-quality fruit is exceptional because it is filtered naturally through the roots, trunk, and branches of the tree, ending in the fruit itself; especially if it's organic.

As mentioned earlier, I highly recommend eating whole fruits. Fruit juice is less ideal, except perhaps during short, targeted detox programs. Whole fruit provides fibre, which slows digestion, reduces the strain on pancreatic beta cells, and prevents sharp spikes in blood sugar. Even though fruit sugars (glucose, fructose, sucrose) are natural and unrefined, they are much gentler when consumed with fibre.

Whole fruits also improve nutrient absorption in the intestines, whereas watery substances like juices are digested too quickly and may bypass full absorption.

The second purest source of water is spring water. True spring water differs from many bottled supermarket waters, which are often processed, stored in plastic, or contain additives. Plastics in particular can leach harmful substances into the water.

Spring water rises naturally from deep layers of the earth, filtered by sand and rock. Sometimes, springs are closer than people think. A quick search may reveal one nearby, allowing you to collect water in glass containers and store it in a cool, shaded place for a couple of weeks of use.

If spring water isn't available, the next best option is filtering tap water to remove sediments, chlorine, fluoride, and heavy metals. Substances like chlorine and bromine; used as disinfectants can disrupt the gut microbiome by harming beneficial bacteria. Fluoride and heavy metals are also toxic at high levels.

Halogens such as fluoride, bromine, and chlorine also compete with iodine, an essential trace nutrient. While tiny amounts of these substances occur naturally in food, the levels added to tap water are far higher than what the body needs.

For this reason, I use an under-sink filter system with three stages: the first for sediments and solids, the second for heavy metals and chlorine, and the third for fluoride. I may include recommendations for filters on my website for those interested.

To wrap up the discussion on hydration: water needs vary based on temperature, climate, age, diet, and activity. While I couldn't find research that gives exact guidelines for people on a natural lifestyle, I've found that those eating naturally develop a stronger connection to their body's signals. They know when they need water and when they've had enough.

Capture 11

Supplements

Supplementation is an important global topic, especially in the Raw Vegan community. This chapter is one I encourage you to read with focus, as proper supplementation is often vital for achieving Ultimate Health.

Do we need to supplement? A short answer is yes. From my experience, a well-structured Raw diet can cover most of our nutritional needs. However, supplements can be necessary depending on factors such as your location, environment, current health condition, and the quality of the raw fruits and vegetables available to you.

Activity level also plays a role: when you are active and consume more food, your nutrient intake rises and may naturally be sufficient. Still, some concerns remain about certain vitamins and minerals. While there are many studies on nutrient deficiencies among vegans, there is limited research specifically addressing Raw Vegans.

It's important to note that Raw Vegan eating differs from a standard vegan diet. Veganism is admirable for its protection of animals and its general health advantages over the Typical Western Diet (T.W.D.). However, many vegan foods are still cooked, which can damage some heat-sensitive nutrients and introduce oxidised compounds. Some vegans also consume processed or "junk" foods, which limits the body's ability to fully heal or efficiently absorb nutrients.

Remember: essential nutrients should ideally be absorbed through your digestive system. Unfortunately, the digestive tract; especially the large intestine (colon) and the liver's metabolic pathways can be affected by unhealthy, processed foods. The colon hosts trillions of beneficial bacteria (the gut flora) that help break down food and support nutrient absorption. Processed foods and toxins disrupt this balance, impairing digestion and reducing the body's ability to absorb vitamins and minerals effectively.

Medication can also damage the colon. Many people take antibacterial tablets (called antibiotics) when they catch a cold or flu or as soon as they feel unwell. While these drugs may kill the harmful bacteria causing the illness, they can also kill the beneficial bacteria in our colon. After damage occurs, and depending on the food intake afterward, colon flora usually takes weeks or even months to recover; sometimes never fully returning to its original diversity.

Cooked food eaters regularly use ingredients with antibacterial properties, such as onions and garlic, which can affect the colon flora to varying degrees. Several studies highlight the health benefits of these ingredients, particularly garlic, which is known for its cholesterol-lowering properties and cardiovascular benefits.

However, this raises the questions: should a healthy body with a natural lifestyle even have high cholesterol levels in the first place? Or cardiovascular diseases? Some Raw Vegans also use garlic, believing that anything raw is beneficial. While garlic has recognised health benefits, it can also slightly disrupt the balance of beneficial gut bacteria in some people and may irritate the digestive tract if used excessively. There are indeed benefits in these raw materials and some medications, but often, their overuse or imbalance can outweigh the benefits.

Based on my research, vitamin and mineral deficiency is a lot more common in everything eaters or people with T.W.D. (specially meat lovers) compared to Raw eaters. I was watching a documentary on the net stating at least 50% of adults in Britain take supplements every day. Are they all vegan or Raw Vegan? Most likely not!

Much research suggests that meat and animal products are rich in proteins and iron, so people who consume meat should generally not have iron deficiencies. However, there are still many individuals on T.W.D. who experience iron deficiencies. For example, I know a person who eats meat almost every day in large quantities and still needs to take iron tablets. When I asked him why he was taking the tablets, he said he had anemia[1], which surprised me because he was eating a lot of meat and animal products weekly. He said it is genetics because his mother was suffering from the same problem.

It is interesting that many diseases in people with a T.W.D. are often attributed by professionals to genetic problems. However, when a person following a plant-based diet becomes iron deficient, their diet is often blamed rather than their genetics. It seems we're sometimes too quick to defend our own habits and question others; instead of recognising that every lifestyle deserves fair and open-minded evaluation.

It is easy to relate any disease or malfunction to genetics (which can be true in some cases). However, we should also consider how we acquire these genes. We inherit them from our parents, who often share the same lifestyle and eating habits as we do. Therefore, it's likely that they experience similar health issues. This connection between genetics and lifestyle is often overlooked.

When discussing supplements, meat lovers often argue, *"Look at those plant-based eaters who still need supplements!"*

---

[1] Anemia is a medical condition in which a person doesn't have enough healthy red blood cells to carry adequate oxygen to their body's tissues. (see Glossary)

But wait a minute; have we considered the millions of people following the Typical Western Diet (T.W.D.) who are suffering because of their dietary choices? How many of them are taking supplements? What diseases do they face? How many die from heart attacks or cancer each day?

The health issues linked to T.W.D. are extensive and serious, yet this criticism is rarely directed toward those eating habits. Perhaps it's time we view all diets with the same level of scrutiny, and focus less on blaming, and more on learning from one another.

In Australia, about 4 million adults live with cardiovascular disease (CVD), and every day, approximately 115 people lose their lives to heart attacks. In the United States, the numbers are far higher, around 18.2 million adults are affected by CVD, with roughly 1,000 people dying from it each day.

Cancer is another major health concern. Each year, more than 140,000 new cases are diagnosed in Australia, and around 50,000 lives are lost to the disease. It's particularly heartbreaking that some of those affected are children.

In the United States, about 40% of the population will face cancer at some stage in their lives, with approximately 600,000 deaths recorded annually. The real number may be even higher when unregistered cases are considered. What's striking is that many of these individuals are not only ordinary people but also top athletes, doctors, and health researchers; a reminder that even knowledge and discipline cannot always protect us from the effects of modern lifestyle and diet.

On another note, you've probably seen plenty of advertising about drinking milk or consuming dairy products such as cheese and yoghurt for their calcium content; promoted as essential for preventing osteoporosis, a condition that leads to bone loss. However, the actual calcium content of milk and dairy products isn't as high as many natural plant foods. For instance, while cow's milk provides about 120–130 mg of calcium per 100 g, yoghurt contains roughly the same amount, while cheese varies widely, ranging between 700 and 1,000 mg per 100 g, depending on the type.

By comparison, several plant foods offer much higher calcium levels: poppy seeds contain around 1,400 mg, sesame seeds about 970 mg, and chia seeds roughly 630 mg per 100 g.

Although calcium content is essential, what's even more important is how well it gets absorbed in our digestive system. As mentioned earlier, one of the main areas affected by the Typical Western Diet (T.W.D.) is the digestive system, particularly the intestines. Many people on this diet experience constipation and sluggish digestion. Milk and dairy products, being low in fibre and sometimes difficult to digest, can further add to intestinal discomfort and worsen constipation in sensitive individuals. When the gut becomes sluggish or inflamed, nutrient absorption; including calcium is reduced.

On the other hand, the consumption of Animal-based and heavily cooked foods can increase the body's acid load, reflected in more acidic urine, which over time may influence mineral balance. pH, which stands for *Potential of Hydrogen*, is a measurement used to determine whether a substance is acidic or alkaline. A pH below 7 is considered acidic, while a pH above 7 is alkaline, and 7 itself is neutral. The human body maintains a slightly alkaline blood pH; typically between **7.35 and 7.45**; and even small deviations from this range can be life-threatening. Therefore, maintaining this delicate balance is as critical to survival as oxygen itself.

In the Typical Western Diet (T.W.D.), milk and dairy products are among the more acidic foods, with milk having a pH between 6.5 and 6.7, yoghurt around 4.3 to 4.4, and cheese between 4.6 and 4.9. Even bread, often considered a healthy food, has a pH of around 5; meaning it contributes to a more acidic system when consumed regularly.

Interestingly, some fruits may taste acidic and have a pH below 7, but they are alkaline-forming after digestion because they produce alkaline byproducts during metabolism. Conversely, animal products, cooked foods, and dairy tend to leave acidic residues ("acid ash") after being metabolised, contributing to the body's overall acid load.

It's also important to understand that the pH scale operates on a **logarithmic** basis; meaning that each whole-number change represents a **tenfold** difference in acidity or alkalinity. For example, a pH of 4 is ten times more acidic than a pH of 5, and one hundred times more acidic than a pH of 6. Conversely, a pH of 9 is ten times more alkaline than a pH of 8. This helps illustrate just how acidic some commonly consumed "health" foods really are.

Additionally, when calcium is dissolved in water, it forms calcium hydroxide ($Ca(OH)_2$), which increases the pH of the solution. A saturated solution of calcium hydroxide typically has a pH around 12–12.5, making it strongly alkaline.

When someone consumes cooked food, meat, and dairy products (most of which have relatively low pH levels) the body works to maintain the blood's natural, slightly alkaline balance. While the blood pH remains tightly regulated between 7.35 and 7.45, some researchers suggest that diets high in acid-forming foods may increase the body's buffering demand, which can influence mineral balance over time. One proposed mechanism is that calcium may be drawn from the bones to help neutralise this acid load, especially when the diet lacks sufficient alkaline-forming foods such as fruits and vegetables.

A person following the Typical Western Diet (T.W.D.) may undergo a blood test showing normal calcium levels, yet a bone density test could reveal reduced bone mass. Interestingly, several large-scale studies have observed that countries with the highest dairy consumption, such as Australia, Norway, Denmark, and the Netherlands, also have some of the highest rates of osteoporosis. This observation challenges the common belief that dairy automatically strengthens bones.

The dairy industry often promotes milk, cheese, and yoghurt as essential sources of calcium for bone health. However, research suggests that bone health depends more on overall diet quality including fruit, vegetable, and mineral intake than on dairy consumption alone. That said, dairy products do contain valuable nutrients, such as protein, calcium, and vitamin B12. My intention is not to dismiss their potential benefits but rather to highlight that they may not always deliver the protective effects often claimed.

Many in the industry may simply be unaware of these nuances, as they too have grown up with the same beliefs. With greater awareness of nutrition and the broader impact of diet on health, even dairy producers might eventually shift toward developing products that better support long-term wellbeing.

Returning to our discussion on supplements, how many examples do we need from people following the Typical Western Diet (T.W.D.) who are already taking supplements? I encourage you to look around; the evidence is everywhere. If you're not one of those on the T.W.D. who takes multivitamins daily, think about the vast number of supplement brands and shelves full of tablets, powders, and fortified foods in supermarkets and pharmacies. Are they all made for vegans or raw eaters? Clearly not. In fact, the largest consumers of supplements are often those who regularly eat meat and dairy.

This raises an important point: who truly needs supplementation the most? Nearly all processed foods today are fortified to replace nutrients lost during industrial processing. Bread, for instance, is enriched with **iron** and **folate**; milk and dairy often contain added vitamin D; table salt is supplemented with iodine; and many breakfast cereals come loaded with synthetic vitamins and minerals.

Even those who claim to eat "pure meat, eggs, and dairy" are indirectly supplementing, since farm animals themselves are routinely given nutritional additives. Farmers do this because they know the soil no longer contains all the minerals required for animal health. Ironically, many people take great care of their livestock's nutrition while overlooking their own.

The widespread need for supplements arises largely from modern farming practices. Continuous cropping and chemical fertilisers have depleted the topsoil, reducing the mineral content of fruits and vegetables. Moreover, most produce is harvested before full ripeness for transport and storage, which further limits nutrient density.

If you've ever grown your own fruits and vegetables organically and allowed them to ripen naturally, you've likely noticed the difference; in taste, texture, and vitality. Such produce not only tastes better but is typically richer in essential nutrients, provided your gut is healthy enough for optimal absorption.

Some health educators claim that supplements aren't necessary. That may be true for those living in pristine conditions, eating ripe, organic fruits straight from the tree under full sunlight. But for most of us, living in cities, under stress, exposed to pollution, and relying on commercial produce, some supplementation can be beneficial and even necessary.

People who follow a natural lifestyle may not consume processed foods or drinks that are fortified with nutrients. Therefore, extra care is needed to ensure the body receives everything it requires.

Within the Raw Vegan community, there's an ongoing discussion about whether supplementation is necessary. Some health professionals advocate for it, while others believe that a well-balanced raw diet can provide everything the body needs.

Many Raw Fruitarian or Raw Vegan advocates believe that fresh fruits, a small number of leafy greens, and some seeds and nuts can supply all essential nutrients, proteins, fats, carbohydrates, vitamins, and minerals, provided they are organic, chemical-free, and eaten fresh. They emphasise that with a healthy raw diet, the gut and absorption system work efficiently, extracting what the body needs. Some even suggest that the body can adapt and synthesise certain compounds from the ingredients we consume and the environment we live in.

Other Raw Vegan experts, however, argue that modern conditions make supplementation important, not because the raw diet is incomplete, but because our environment and food sources have changed. Today's processed and fortified foods often compensate for depleted nutrients in the soil or lost during transport and storage, and raw eaters avoid these artificially enriched products.

Both perspectives carry truth. The necessity for supplementation depends on many factors, including where you live, what you eat, your genetics, health condition, stress levels, and activity. Thousands of years ago, humans living in tropical environments under the sun, surrounded by fresh, nutrient-rich fruit and pure air, likely didn't need supplements. But our world today is very different. We face pollution, stress, artificial light, radio frequencies, and chemically altered food systems, all of which can deplete our nutrient stores and increase our needs.

The agricultural industry, while essential, is not focused on human nutrition as its main goal. Farmers often aim for yield, size, colour, and shelf life rather than nutrient density. Continuous cropping, soil depletion, and the use of fertilisers and chemicals mean that fruits and vegetables may not contain the same nutrition they once did. Additionally, premature harvesting and long transport times reduce vitamin and mineral levels before food reaches our tables.

For example, studies have shown significant variation in vitamin content between produce grown in different regions. One analysis of oranges across the USA found that some contained as little as 10% of the Vitamin C expected based on food composition tables. Storage conditions can also degrade nutrients; exposure to fluorescent or LED light can destroy over 60% of Vitamin C in fruit.

Our bodies are remarkable but still rely on dietary sources for essential nutrients. The nine essential amino acids must come from food, as the body cannot synthesise them. Likewise, vitamin K1 must be ingested before the body converts it to K2, and minerals can only be absorbed if they exist in the soil or water where our food grows.

I once knew a family in far north Queensland- Australia, living simply on fresh, local fruits, much of it grown on their land or foraged from the wild, and avoiding all chemicals and processed products. They reported thriving on this natural lifestyle without any supplements. But how many of us can live under such ideal conditions? For most people today, supplementation is not a sign of failure, it's a practical necessity to compensate for environmental and agricultural limitations. It helps ensure our bodies receive what they need to function optimally and to minimise the risk of deficiency or long-term illness.

Growing your own food is one of the best ways to ensure access to fresh, nutrient-rich produce. Even if you live in an apartment, there are plenty of creative options, such as container gardens, vertical gardens, or hydroponic systems. Online resources, including YouTube tutorials, can guide you step-by-step regardless of space or experience. When you grow your own food, you control the entire process, from soil quality to ripeness, guaranteeing it's organic, chemical-free, and handled with care.

If you have access to local farms, another great option is to pick produce directly from the source or buy from farmers' markets, where fruits and vegetables are often fresher and naturally ripened. Whenever possible, choose organic produce that's fully matured, as ripening increases nutrient content and flavour.

Some people ask how they can afford organic food. My answer is simple: compare it to what's already being spent on medications, energy drinks, and short-term indulgences like alcohol, coffee, or processed snacks. Many of us spend far more on temporary comforts than on long-term health. Investing in your health pays dividends, fewer hospital visits, less medication, more energy, and, most importantly, time saved from illness and recovery. When viewed through that lens, organic food becomes a valuable investment rather than an expense.

As we've discussed, nutrition is deeply personal. Factors such as age, genetics, environment, lifestyle, stress, and activity level all play a role. Conducting your own research and having an annual comprehensive blood test reviewed by a qualified practitioner can help identify what your body truly needs. Keep in mind that not all vitamins and minerals are routinely measured, so remain proactive and informed.

Mental and emotional well-being also influence how well your body absorbs and utilises nutrients. Chronic stress, for instance, increases the body's demand for certain vitamins and minerals. A balanced approach; combining proper diet, physical activity, rest, and mental clarity forms the foundation for what I call *Ultimate Health*.

In short, a diet rich in fruits, complemented by some vegetables, nuts, and seeds, can provide nearly all the essential nutrients your body needs with only a few exceptions that we'll explore in the following section.

Critical Nutrition

The carbohydrates, proteins, fats, vitamins, and minerals we've discussed so far are the foundation of human nutrition. You can obtain nearly all the nutrients your body needs from a wide variety of fresh fruits, especially tropical ones along with leafy greens, nuts, and seeds.

While managing carbohydrates, proteins, and fats can be straightforward, there are a few other nutrients that deserve extra attention. These are the ones you must actively monitor in your diet or source from reputable, ideally Raw Vegan supplements when necessary.

Please note these nutrients are critical for everyone, not only for those following a natural lifestyle. Even individuals on a Typical Western Diet (T.W.D.) often experience deficiencies in key nutrients such as iron, vitamin B12, and iodine. According to global research, vitamin D deficiency affects more than half of the world's population, regardless of diet or geography, largely due to limited sun exposure and modern indoor lifestyles.

These essential nutrients must come from external sources through diet, sunlight, or supplementation to support optimal health, hormone production, and cellular repair. In the following sections, I'll explain each of these critical nutrients in detail based on my research, experience, and practical understanding. Still, it's important to conduct your own research, consult your health professional, and consider personalised advice based on your unique health needs.

Vitamin B12

Vitamin B12 is a fascinating topic in the vegan and Raw Vegan communities, and one of the most misunderstood. It's often raised by experts and followers of the Typical Western Diet (T.W.D.) as the main reason to discourage people from adopting a plant-based or natural lifestyle.

Vitamin B12 has two important aspects; how we obtain it from external sources, and how efficiently our body can absorb and utilise it. Interestingly, even many people on the T.W.D. who consume large quantities of animal products; theoretically rich in B12; are still deficient, usually because of impaired digestion and poor intestinal absorption.

Vitamin B12, also known as cobalamin, is a water-soluble vitamin crucial for various bodily functions, including cell formation. It plays essential roles in producing red blood cells, synthesising DNA, forming nerves and crucial for brain functions.

Although most water-soluble vitamins aren't stored for long, B12 and B9 (folate) are exceptions. Folate is stored for only a few days, but B12 can be stored in the liver for several years; sometimes up to a decade.

Since we need less than 3 µg (microgram)[1] a day, deficiency often develops slowly and may not appear in blood tests until years after dietary intake stops. Still, untreated deficiency can lead to anaemia and nerve damage, which can be permanent.

Typically, our body doesn't retain water-soluble vitamins, necessitating daily intake. However, there are two exceptions: Vitamin B9 (Folate) and B12, which our liver can store them. While both can be stored in the liver, folate is stored for a very short term, whereas B12 is typically stored for much longer periods.

For B12 to be absorbed in the small intestine, the stomach must produce a protein called the intrinsic factor. Without it, even high dietary intake may not help. Animal products naturally contain B12, and some processed foods are fortified with it. However, where should we get our B12 if we remove animal products and fortified processed foods?

Let's first explore how animals obtain their B12. As the name *cobalamin* suggests, its key component is cobalt, a trace metal found in soil. B12 is synthesised by microorganisms that use cobalt. Animals such as cows eat unwashed grass containing these bacteria, allowing them to obtain B12 naturally. They also host beneficial intestinal bacteria that help maintain their B12 levels.

Due to the depletion of cobalt in the Earth's topsoil, farm animals today are often given B12-fortified feed. Farmers generally prioritise the health of their animals to ensure proper growth and milk production.

---

[1] Some sources refer to 7 µg per day.

People on the T.W.D. get B12 either directly from animal products or indirectly from fortified foods. When you follow a natural lifestyle, you don't consume either, so you no longer take B12 indirectly through the food chain.

It also appears that when humans began relying on animal products, our bodies gradually lost the ability to produce B12 independently, as it was consistently supplied through food. There are, however, Raw Vegans with natural lifestyles who don't take B12 supplements yet still maintain healthy levels. From my understanding, every food that contains other B vitamins, such as B3 and B9, also carries trace amounts of cobalt. A healthy body with a balanced intestine, functional colon flora, and adequate intrinsic factor may eventually learn to produce some B12 from available cobalt. This process can take years and differs from person to person, and in some, it may not occur at all.

So, what should you do? First, get a blood test to check your B12 level. Choose a modern test that measures the *active form* of B12, or ask for an **MMA** (Methylmalonic Acid) test, which is even more accurate. MMA levels rise in the blood and urine when B12 is low. You may need to take B12 supplements depending on your results. In severe cases, often in long-term vegans or vegetarians, injections may be needed. Otherwise, sublingual tablets work well. Many use the **methylcobalamin** form, which is active and easily absorbed. Some are chewable and designed to dissolve under the tongue; avoid eating or drinking until fully absorbed, usually within 30 minutes. You can start with one tablet daily and adjust based on follow-up tests every six to twelve months.

Another form, **cyanocobalamin**, contains a small cyanide component and must be converted in the body before use. It's less efficiently absorbed, so I don't recommend it. Methylcobalamin is safer, more active, and better retained.

If your body doesn't produce enough B12 naturally, long-term supplementation may be necessary; and that's perfectly fine. It's far better to prevent deficiency and protect your nerves and energy levels than to risk it.

Iodine

The second essential and critical nutrient, which is rare in the soil, is iodine.

You may have heard that iodine is vital for the function of the thyroid gland, a key organ that regulates body metabolism. However, iodine is not only important for the thyroid; it is required by all tissues and cells throughout the body, as well as for a strong immune system.

The Thymus gland[1] needs iodine and selenium to produce T-cells[2], which play a crucial role in destroying abnormal or cancerous cells. Selenium is another critical nutrient explained later.

Medical science has recognised iodine deficiency for many decades. To combat this, iodised salt was introduced in the early 1900s. You may remember (or have heard of) goiter, an enlarged thyroid gland that used to be common, particularly in women, who typically require more iodine.

The thyroid produces the hormones T3 (triiodothyronine) and T4 (thyroxine), which are essential for weight control, muscle strength, nervous system balance, and maintaining body

---

[1] A very important gland part of the lymph system.

[2] T-cells, a type of lymphocyte, are produced in the bone marrow as part of the white blood cells and mature in the thymus gland.

temperature. It is the most efficient organ at concentrating iodine and is its biggest consumer. However, iodine is also needed by every cell in the body, not just the thyroid; a fact that is often overlooked.

When dietary iodine is insufficient, the body prioritises the thyroid and sends most of the available iodine there. Goiter occurs as the thyroid enlarges in an effort to capture more iodine and maintain normal hormone production. The numbers 3 and 4 in T3 and T4 refer to the number of iodine atoms in each molecule; so when iodine is scarce, these hormones cannot be produced in sufficient amounts. Based on my research and discussions with doctors, it seems that the medical field often underestimates iodine's broader role and the optimal intake levels required for whole-body sufficiency.

In the early 20th century, governments in developed nations added small amounts of iodine to table salt to prevent severe deficiencies such as goiter and related developmental issues. The current Recommended Daily Intake (RDI) is about 150 µg (micrograms), which is enough to prevent goiter but may not be sufficient for full-body iodine saturation. Other organs including the thymus, breasts, ovaries, prostate, and even the brain also require iodine to function properly.

It is often reported that the Japanese consume between 1 and 3 milligrams of iodine per day, primarily from seaweed and other marine plants; an intake that is dozens of times higher than the Recommended Dietary Intake (RDI) set by the World Health Organization (WHO). This naturally high iodine consumption is believed to contribute to Japan's historically low rates of iodine deficiency and the disorders associated with insufficient intake.

However, research also shows that excessive iodine intake can lead to its own set of thyroid-related problems, and some iodine-induced conditions are more common in certain Japanese populations as a result of their very high consumption.

Fresh seaweed is among the best natural sources of iodine, but care must be taken: seaweed grown in shallow or polluted waters can accumulate heavy metals such as arsenic, lead, or cadmium. Brown seaweeds; particularly kelp and hijiki tend to accumulate more of these toxins, so the source and quality are critical. Consuming seaweed in moderation and choosing products from trusted suppliers is important to avoid contamination risks.

Iodine is a volatile trace element and can evaporate or degrade through sublimation, meaning that dried seaweed or cooked seafood (as in the Typical Western Diet, T.W.D.) often contains much less iodine than expected.

As mentioned earlier, many medical practitioners are not deeply familiar with testing or correcting iodine deficiency, and very few laboratories conduct specialised iodine tests. After extensive research, I found a testing laboratory in Melbourne- Australia for measuring iodine. I highly recommend consulting a qualified practitioner who understands iodine metabolism and can guide you through proper testing and supplementation if required.

Iodine works synergistically with other nutrients; especially selenium; so balancing these is vital for safety and effectiveness. Correcting iodine levels requires expertise and should not be done without professional supervision, as both deficiency and excess can be harmful.

To conclude, iodine deficiency can affect anyone, regardless of diet. However, people following a natural or raw lifestyle, who typically avoid iodised table salt, dairy, and animal products may be at higher risk and should monitor their iodine status carefully.

I recommend checking the label of any supplement and seaweed products and ensuring that your total daily iodine intake does not exceed approximately 650 µg, unless advised otherwise by a qualified healthcare professional. This level is generally considered safe for most people and helps reduce the risk of thyroid disruption from excessive intake.

Vitamin D

Vitamin D, a fat-soluble group of vitamins, is another critical nutrient important for absorbing calcium, magnesium, and phosphate, which are essential for bone health, the immune system, and cardiovascualr health. There is growing awareness in the community about the importance of Vitamin D. Yet, it has been often neglected by many people, including me, and before starting my natural lifestyle.

You may be surprised to know that many people around the world are Vitamin D deficient. Regardless of your diet and lifestyle you might be Vitamin D deficient if you do not address it properly. You may have also heard how important Vitamin D is for your immune system, preventing cancer cell growth, controlling infections, and reducing inflammation.

Naturally, Vitamin D is produced by our bodies using cholesterol and UV rays from the sun, but it can also be supplied through oral supplementation. The Vitamin D deficiency pandemic began when humans became more civilised, migrated from tropical environments with abundant sunshine to colder, cloud-covered areas, and spent most of their time indoors, mainly in front of screens, forgetting about outdoor living. Even when outdoors, we often cover our skin to avoid sunburn or apply sunscreen, which limits UVB penetration. As a result, the skin produces less Vitamin D, even in sunny climates.

Those following the T.W.D. may obtain small amounts from foods such as fish, egg yolks, or sunlight-exposed wild mushrooms, as well as fortified cereals and milk. Yet, these sources generally provide only enough to prevent severe deficiency (such as rickets[1]) rather than to maintain optimal levels for whole-body health.

Public concern about skin cancer has also contributed to reduced sun exposure. While protecting the skin from burning is important[2], moderate sunlight remains essential for Vitamin D production. Some research (see references) has observed that rates of skin cancer have continued to rise despite widespread sunscreen use, though this link is complex and influenced by many factors. Certain chemical ingredients in sunscreens may also irritate the skin (some contain ingredients like nanoparticles that can penetrate the skin, acting as external toxins and potentially contributing to the development of cancerous cells), and excessive UV avoidance can inadvertently lower Vitamin D levels, which is essential for the immune system to protect the body.

Many people use oral Vitamin D supplements, which can help restore or maintain adequate levels. However, the body's natural production through UVB exposure is generally more efficient and self-regulated. Because Vitamin D is fat-soluble, it is stored in the liver and fatty tissue, allowing for long-term use but also creating a risk of toxicity if taken in excess. Very high doses may cause

---

[1] Rickets is a medical condition that affects bone development usually in children, leading to soft and weak bones.

[2] There are connections between sunburn and skin cancers, and skin protection is required most of the time.

hypercalcemia (elevated blood calcium), leading to nausea, fatigue, or, in rare cases, kidney complications.

When produced naturally from sunlight, the body creates precisely what it needs no more, no less. This finely balanced system supports all tissues and avoids the risk of overdose. Individual Vitamin D requirements vary depending on factors such as age, body composition, skin tone, location, health status, and the body's ability to convert Vitamin D into its active form (Vitamin D_3). This means that a single daily recommendation cannot suit everyone. This should help you understand why oral supplementation may not be as efficient as exposure to UVB rays.

Sunlight exposure also stimulates the production of other beneficial compounds in the skin:

- **Vitamin D sulfate**
- **Cholesterol sulfate,**
- **Beta-endorphin, and**
- **Nitric oxide**

You might not have heard of them before, but they play significant roles in maintaining health. You may ask why these nutrients are important. Based on my research and understanding, their complete roles are still not fully known from a scientific standpoint, but there are some important notes worth mentioning.

The Vitamin D sulphate is a water-soluble counterpart to the fat-soluble version of Vitamin D, which is usually supplemented. As a water-soluble form, Vitamin D sulfate can easily travel through the bloodstream and nourish cells throughout the body. This highlights its importance for optimal health, as it can move freely around the body, unlike the fat-soluble form of Vitamin D. Unfortunately, it cannot be supplemented, or it is better to say currently there is no supplement for D-sulphate in the market.

Another important nutrient the body produces in the presence of UVB is cholesterol sulfate. While the full function of cholesterol sulfate, which is part of the cell membrane, is not yet fully understood by scientists, it is believed to act as a stabiliser. It does this by generating a negatively charged field around cells, preventing them from sticking together and facilitating the smooth movement of blood through tiny capillaries, which is important for cardiovascular health.

The other important compounds produced in our skin by UVB exposure are beta-endorphins, which are feel-good hormones that also act as neurotransmitters. Have you noticed that you feel good when you wake up on a lovely sunny day and expose yourself to sunlight? This may be partly because beta-endorphins are released, enhancing your mood. This could explain why many people enjoy and sometimes feel a strong desire to expose their skin to the sun on the beach on a nice sunny day.

This sunbathing desire is mainly driven by the production of these wonderful feel-good hormones.

Sunshine, specifically UVB rays, also helps the skin produce nitric oxide (NO- or nitrogen monoxide), which is important for skin health and preventing wrinkles and lines. Nitric oxide also helps regulate blood pressure, reducing the risk of cardiovascular diseases (CVD) and helping protect tissues from damage due to a low blood supply. A lack of sufficient sunshine can be a significant factor in the increase of heart attacks during winter for people living far from the equator.

After considering all the above and the importance of daily sunshine, you may ask how much sunshine you need and how you can tell if the sunshine is strong enough to produce all the necessary nutrients in your skin, correct? Well, these are million-dollar questions, but the answer is not straightforward. It depends on where you live, the altitude, the UV index, your skin type, and the time of day you have a chance to expose your skin to the sun.

You should appreciate how complicated this can be. The first thing you should consider is ensuring you do not burn your skin as any form of skin burn damages tissue and increases health risks.

You will need to do your own research, but based on my findings, about 5 to 15 minutes of sun exposure per day is generally sufficient when the sun's position in the sky means your shadow is shorter than your height. Fair skin usually requires less time, while darker skin typically needs longer exposure. Keep in mind that there are additional factors that require consideration.

What if you live far from the equator and there are no sunny days during winter or even other times of the year)? How can you get daily sunshine when there is no sunshine at all? Well, you have two options: take an oral Vitamin D supplement or buy a phototherapy device that emits UVB-simulating light. The first option is good for the short term and until you can purchase the device or get a chance to expose your skin to the sun.

There are some good oral vegan Vitamin D supplements available, which you should take after getting your Vitamin D levels tested under the supervision of a health practitioner.

Based on your budget, you can then buy a Vitamin D lamp and follow the instructions to ensure you get enough daily UVB. This will help your body not only produce Vitamin D but also synthesise other essential nutrients mentioned above, which are crucial for your Ultimate Health.

I had been taking oral Vitamin D supplements for some time until I bought a UVB lamp (a Vitamin D lamp). I noticed a significant improvement and my Vitamin D levels are now within the optimal range. I will most likely introduce some resources for these lamps on my website, should you be interested in considering them.

Vitamin E

Vitamin E is another critical nutrient for overall health. It plays an especially important role in maintaining healthy skin, eyes, and immune function.

Vitamin E is a fat-soluble antioxidant that helps protect cells from damage caused by free radicals, unstable molecules formed during normal metabolism when the body converts food into energy. Free radicals can also arise from external sources, such as air pollution, cigarette smoke, and ultraviolet (UV) light from the sun. Heating or burning food can generate additional oxidative compounds that increase the free-radical load on the body.

Vitamin E exists in **eight natural forms**; four tocopherols and four tocotrienols; each with alpha, beta, gamma, and delta variants. Among them, **alpha-tocopherol** is the most biologically active form in humans.

Vitamin E contributes to:

- Protecting cells and tissues from oxidative stress
- Supporting the immune system
- Maintaining healthy skin and vision
- Assisting in the formation of red blood cells

Deficiency, though uncommon, can lead to symptoms such as weakened immunity, muscle and nerve problems, or vision changes.

Contrary to common belief, Vitamin E deficiency can occur in anyone, not just those on restrictive diets, especially when dietary fat intake is very low or when fresh produce is limited.

For those following a natural or raw lifestyle, Vitamin E can be obtained from creamy tropical fruits such as avocado, durian, papaya, mango, and blackberries. However, because Vitamin E is fat-soluble, moderation is important, especially when relying on higher-fat foods like avocados or seeds.

Good plant sources include:

- Kiwi fruit, a refreshing, lower-fat option rich in Vitamin E.

- Almonds and sunflower seeds, excellent sources, though they also contain higher levels of omega-6 fatty acids, which should be balanced with omega-3 sources.

Since fat-soluble vitamins can accumulate in the body, supplementation should only be considered under professional supervision. Obtaining Vitamin E from natural, whole foods remains the safest and most effective approach.

As always, it's wise to review your diet and do your own research to ensure you're meeting your daily needs for this essential vitamin.

Zinc

Zinc is another essential trace mineral that can sometimes be challenging to obtain in a Raw Fruitarian (Raw Vegan) diet, though this can also affect people following the Typical Western Diet (T.W.D.) or other eating patterns.

One reason is that many modern agricultural soils are low in zinc, as it's rarely replenished during fertilisation. Plants grown in such soil, and the animals that eat them, may therefore have lower zinc content.

Zinc plays a vital role in many bodily processes, including:

- Supporting a healthy immune system
- Promoting wound healing
- Aiding cell growth and repair
- Regulating hormones, including insulin and reproductive hormones
- Supporting normal growth and development in children

Some nuts and seeds contain moderate amounts of zinc, for example, pumpkin seeds, hemp seeds, cashews, and sesame seeds though their absorption can be reduced by the presence of phytates, naturally occurring compounds that bind minerals. Soaking or sprouting seeds and nuts can help improve zinc availability.

Unfortunately, accurately measuring zinc levels can be difficult, as standard blood tests often reflect only short-term zinc status. For this reason, many people rely on symptoms to gauge possible deficiency, such as:

- Slow wound healing

- Reduced appetite

- Hair thinning

- Changes in taste or smell

When reliable testing isn't available, it's important to monitor how your body feels and responds.

If supplementation becomes necessary, look for high-quality vegan-friendly forms, such as zinc gluconate, zinc citrate, or liquid ionic zinc. Personally, I've found that liquid zinc and Raw Vegan tablets work effectively, but it's always best to research thoroughly and discuss your choice with a qualified health practitioner before starting any supplement.

Selenium

Selenium plays an essential role in many bodily functions.

It is required for DNA production, thyroid hormone metabolism, and immune system function, and it helps protect cells from oxidative damage caused by free radicals. Selenium works closely with iodine to support the lymphatic and immune systems, particularly through the thymus gland, which uses both minerals to produce T-cells; the white blood cells responsible for identifying and destroying abnormal or cancerous cells.

Selenium is also important for heart health. Severe deficiency can lead to a rare condition known as Keshan disease, a form of cardiomyopathy that may result in heart failure. Other possible symptoms of selenium deficiency include hair loss, muscle weakness, and mental fatigue or "fog."

The richest known food source of selenium is the Brazil nut. In some regions, eating just one nut a day can provide the recommended daily intake. However, selenium content varies widely depending on the mineral levels in the soil where the trees grow. In areas with selenium-poor soil, the nuts may contain far less of this nutrient.

Because selenium is needed only in trace amounts, excess intake can cause toxicity. For that reason, supplementation should be approached carefully. The safe upper limit for adults is around 400 µg per day, and most people need only 55 µg daily.

As always, it's best to research your options, discuss them with a trusted health professional, and consider a reliable, vegan-friendly supplement only if needed.

Magnesium

Magnesium is the last critical trace element I want to highlight, and it is another essential mineral that supports hundreds of biochemical reactions in the body. It's often called the "relaxation mineral" because of its calming effects on muscles, nerves, and even the mind.

Magnesium plays a vital role in:

- Supporting energy production and the function of enzymes
- Maintaining muscle and nerve function, helping prevent cramps and spasms
- Regulating heart rhythm and blood pressure
- Contributing to bone health by working alongside calcium and vitamin D
- Supporting sleep quality and the body's ability to manage stress

Unfortunately, magnesium deficiency is common across all diets not just among Raw Vegans. Modern agricultural practices have gradually depleted magnesium from the soil, and processed foods in the Typical Western Diet (T.W.D.) remove much of what little magnesium remains. Even those eating plenty of fruits and vegetables may fall short if the soil in their region is low in this mineral.

Symptoms of mild magnesium deficiency may include:

- **Muscle twitches or cramps**

- **Fatigue or weakness**

- **Mood changes such as anxiety or irritability**

- **Poor sleep or restlessness**

- **Irregular heartbeat in more severe cases**

For Raw Vegans, the best natural sources of magnesium include leafy greens, avocados, figs, bananas, and soaked nuts and seeds, especially pumpkin seeds and almonds. Soaking nuts and seeds also helps reduce compounds that interfere with its absorption.

If you still experience symptoms or your diet is limited, a high-quality vegan magnesium supplement may help. Forms such as magnesium glycinate, magnesium citrate, or magnesium malate tend to be well absorbed and gentle on the stomach. As always, check your levels through a blood test and discuss supplementation with your health practitioner.

My Feast

We've already discussed how an unbalanced diet can harm health and contribute to various illnesses. In this chapter, I'll share my personal lifestyle; what I eat and how I structure my day to minimise the risk of sickness and maintain vitality.

However, please note that this is my personal choice, not a prescription or recommendation. Everyone's needs differ depending on their genetics, activity level, environment, and available foods. Use this simply as an example to inspire your own exploration, guided by research, your health practitioner, and your dietitian.

Main foods

As a fully Raw Vegan, my everyday food comprises around:

- **80% fruits,**
- **10% veggies,**
- **10% seeds, legumes and nuts**

I usually wake up between 4:30 and 5:00 a.m. and drink two glasses of warm filtered water. This gently prepares my digestive system for elimination and hydration. Around this time, I also take my main supplement tablet (mostly B12). Sometimes I enjoy a glass of fresh coconut water, directly from a coconut, not the packaged kind.

If you're in a detox phase, especially during the first two weeks, a simple glass of lemon or lime water in the morning can help. To prepare it, squeeze fresh juice into filtered room-temperature water and drink it slowly within five minutes, as lemon juice oxidises quickly and loses much of its vitamin C when exposed to air.

Before noon, I usually have meals made of seasonal fruits. During winter, I usually enjoy a plate of citrus fruits, while in summer, I prefer berries, watermelon, or pears. Fresh, seasonal fruit is essential to me, as it provides maximum energy, hydration, and nutrition.

Later in the day, I usually have my main smoothie, made from chia seeds, hemp seeds, sun-dried raisins, a small amount of black unhulled sesame seeds, dates, and my green powders. This combination delivers a broad and balanced range of nutrients. I typically soak the seeds and raisins overnight and keep the mixture refrigerated.

Throughout the day, I enjoy a variety of fruits such as strawberries, blueberries, persimmons, loquats, pomegranates, apples, custard apples, cherries, kiwis, and peaches, depending on availability and season.

In the afternoon, I choose denser and starchier fruits that digest more slowly, pineapple (if I can find ripe ones), bananas, papayas, dates, figs, jujubes, and raisins. When available, sapotes and durian are wonderful additions.

In the evening, sometimes I prepare a nourishing meal made from sprouted lentils, chickpeas, and quinoa, mixed with shredded carrot and a quarter of an avocado. For dressing, I use only freshly squeezed lemon or lime juice. This simple yet delicious dish provides a wide range of nutrients, B-vitamins, vitamin C, choline, vitamins K, A, E, and minerals such as iron, magnesium, potassium, and zinc plus fibre and beneficial plant compounds like carotenoids and polyphenols. Sometimes, instead of this mix, I prepare a salad of leafy greens using the same dressing.

Occasionally I include a small amount of nuts in my diet, typically Brazil nuts, walnuts, hazelnuts, almonds, and pistachios. I soak them for about 24 hours before eating to "activate" them. This activation process mimics germination, awakening enzymes and making the nuts easier to digest and absorb. Soaking also rehydrates the nuts and reduces certain natural inhibitors such as phytates, further improving nutrient availability.

To clarify, salads and nuts make up less than 20 % of my overall diet. My primary focus is on fresh fruits, which form the majority of my daily intake. All the foods I eat are raw, unheated, mostly organic, and kept as close to their natural state as possible. I consider myself fortunate to have access to such fresh, high-quality produce and supplements daily.

During mango season, I sometimes make a mango or banana smoothie for my evening meal. Alongside, I include my main supplement raw, organic barley-grass juice powder. It's dried under nitrogen to prevent oxidation and preserve delicate trace minerals such as chromium, molybdenum, copper, and iron, along with heat-sensitive vitamins.

To further balance my Omega-3 and Omega-6 intake and ensure I receive essential amino acids, I often add a small amount of ground chia seed and hemp seed to my smoothie. Occasionally, I combine chia seeds with sesame seeds, sunflower seeds, or pepitas for variety and added nutrition. Sometimes, I blend them with papaya and figs for a richer texture and taste.

I typically listen to the signals I receive from my body for when to eat or drink. I usually feel genuine hunger every two to three hours, and I let that guide me naturally.

I also follow the practice of eating one type of fruit per meal and avoiding the mixing of too many varieties. Occasionally, I combine fruits from the same category such as different berries or melons, but generally, I find that simpler combinations work best for digestion.

Fruits have distinct structures, enzymes, and digestion times. When mixed in large variety, they can linger longer in the digestive system, sometimes leading to mild fermentation and discomfort, such as bloating or gas, especially in sensitive individuals. Keeping fruit combinations simple usually supports smoother digestion and more efficient nutrient absorption.

There are various fruit-combination guidelines available that you can explore, and I plan to include some on my website. One widely recognised principle, for example, is to avoid mixing melons with other fruits, as they digest much faster than most others.

It's worth mentioning that people sometimes ask me about Eskimos or Inuits, who live in Alaska and other Arctic regions where access to fruits and vegetables is extremely limited. They point out that the Inuit diet is predominantly animal-based, rich in fat and protein, and that these populations have been reported to experience lower rates of heart disease and some chronic conditions traditionally linked to the Typical Western Diet (T.W.D.).

It's true that very cold climates offer few fruit options, and humans who settled there had to adapt to what nature provided. Science suggests humans first evolved in Africa, a tropical environment, not in cold regions. As opportunistic creatures, our ancestors began exploring other places to live.

They adapted to the new climate and conditions, but this adaptation does not necessarily mean they lived in their optimal health. For example, when someone starts smoking, their body quickly adapts to the toxins from the cigarette. Does their body get hurt by the smoke? You should know the answer. Similarly, our body can adapt to various conditions as a survival mechanism, but this does not mean we can maintain good health with any diet and food intake.

While Eskimos may have limited fruit options, they still consume some berries, seaweed, and plants. Lichens and moss, which are vegetables, also grow in the Arctic. The active Inuit community eats fish and raw meat, consuming the whole animal without cooking, unlike those with a Typical Western Diet (T.W.D.).

This diet provides them with energy and essential nutrients from raw materials. However, due to the lack of sufficient fruits and vegetables, they age quickly and rarely live beyond 60 years, according to my research.

Returning to the main topic, the foods and principles I've shared are simply what I've found to support my own Ultimate Health and physical performance. I encourage you to do your own research and discover what works best for your individual health, environment, and body.

My Supplements

As a Raw Vegan, my main fuel comes from raw, ripe, sweet, seasonal, and unprocessed fruits in their purest form. I usually eat about two to three kilograms of fruit daily, along with some vegetables, seeds, and nuts. These include seasonal fruits, dried fruits, soaked chia seeds, hemp seeds, Brazil nuts, walnuts, hazelnuts, pistachios, almonds, pepitas, sunflower seeds, and sprouted quinoa, lentils, mung beans, and chickpeas, all natural, unsalted, and raw.

I soak or sprout most seeds, nuts, and legumes for about 24 hours to activate their enzymes, reduce phytates, and make them easier to digest and more bioavailable.

Occasionally, I include seaweed, kelp, chlorella, and spirulina in powdered, raw, and organic form. These are excellent sources of trace minerals, particularly iodine (from kelp) and other essential elements. I also take about 1–2 tablespoons of raw organic barley grass juice powder daily, usually in a smoothie. It provides rare micronutrients and vitamins such as A, E, and K, several B-group vitamins, and minerals including iron, manganese, molybdenum, copper, chromium, and magnesium.

For Vitamin D, I use a phototherapy device during winter when sunshine is limited.

Because fruit and vegetable intake alone may not supply all the nutrients needed for optimal function, I complement my diet with a few vegan supplements, including essential fatty acids, vitamins, and minerals. I take a vegan Omega-3 oil derived from algae grown in controlled tanks, free from ocean contaminants. These provide DHA and EPA critical for brain, eye, and heart health as well as support for protein synthesis and cell structure.

I also take a vegan multivitamin on occasion to cover nutrients that are lower in my fruit supply and a magnesium tablet before bed to support relaxation and muscle recovery.

I want to emphasise that everything I've shared here is based on my personal experience. This is not a recommendation or dietary prescription. You should research thoroughly, consult your health practitioner or dietitian, and make informed decisions based on your own health, environment, and available foods. Ultimately, you are responsible for your own wellbeing, and the best choices come from knowledge and self-awareness.

Processing

I consume most of my food in its natural, unprocessed state. However, I've noticed that some Raw Vegans rely heavily on food preparation methods such as juicing, dehydrating, mixing, and blending.

While occasional processing can fit within a Raw diet, it may not be the best long-term practice for achieving Ultimate Health, especially if done frequently. I recommend keeping processed meals to no more than one or two per day, focusing primarily on whole, unaltered fruits and vegetables.

If you choose to diversify your meals with some processing, consider the following points.

Minimise Fruit Juicing

There are three main reasons why excessive juicing may not be ideal.

1. Oxidation and Nutrient Loss. Juicing exposes the internal parts of fruits to oxygen, which leads to rapid oxidation and a reduction in certain nutrients, especially Vitamin C, one of the most oxygen-sensitive vitamins.

2. Rapid Sugar Absorption. Most fruits contain natural sugars, primarily glucose and fructose, that are easy for the body to use as energy and far safer than refined sugars. However, eating whole fruit provides fibre, which slows down sugar absorption and ensures a smoother release of glucose into the bloodstream. This reduces strain on the pancreas by preventing sudden insulin spikes

and helps the liver process fructose more efficiently. In contrast, juice lacks fibre, causing quicker sugar absorption and less satiety.

3. Higher Sugar Concentration. When juicing, it's easy to consume more fruit than you would eat whole. For example, a single glass of orange juice may require five or six oranges, whereas you might only eat two or three in one sitting. This increases total sugar intake unnecessarily. The lack of fibre also means you may feel less full, encouraging larger servings.

That said, fruit-juice fasting can sometimes be used therapeutically to support detoxification or recovery from certain health conditions. When done under professional supervision and for a limited time, short juice fasts can help rest the digestive system and deliver concentrated nutrients. However, they should not replace regular meals or become a long-term practice, as whole fruits provide superior nutrition and digestive balance.

If you do enjoy juice, try to retain some pulp to restore fibre content, and drink it soon after preparation to minimise oxidation and nutrient loss.

Making Smoothies

Instead of fruit juice, I recommend having smoothies, which retain the fruit's natural fibre. However, it's important to know which fruits can be combined, as not all make good companions. I plan to provide a list of compatible fruit combinations on my website, but here are a few examples:

A mix of bananas and dates makes an excellent, energy-rich smoothie. During mango season, a mango and date smoothie is another delicious option. Fresh figs, or soaked dried figs (soaked for 24 hours) combined with dates also make a tasty and nutritious blend.

Instead of using a mechanical blender, which can slightly warm the ingredients and increase oxidation, you can simply mash or mix the fruit with a fork. I often grind chia seeds, hemp seeds, and occasionally sunflower seeds and add them to my smoothies for extra nutrients. Sometimes I sprinkle raw organic coconut flakes on top for flavour, texture, and a small boost of Omega-9.

When making smoothies, I suggest leaving some small fruit pieces in the mix. This encourages light chewing, which, as mentioned in the *How to Eat* chapter, supports better digestion and nutrient absorption.

Drink your smoothie slowly and mindfully, but avoid taking too long, as smoothies can oxidise quickly. It's best to make them fresh and consume them immediately rather than storing them in the fridge for later. You'll notice the colour darkening over time, even under refrigeration; a clear sign of oxidation and nutrient loss.

Mixing Fat and Sugar

There are quite a few studies suggesting not mixing fat and sugar, such as making smoothies from fruits and nuts combined. The main argument is that these two are only found separately in nature. Additionally, our body needs to release insulin to process sugar, while fat creates resistance against insulin, leading to digestive problems and putting pressure on internal organs such as the pancreas.

On the other hand, some fruits contain natural fats, especially creamy fruits that grow in tropical conditions, which are biologically well-suited for human consumption.

From my research, when combined with naturally sweet fruits, these natural fats may not cause digestive issues. For example, most of the time I make my smoothies with chia and hemp seeds and do not experience any digestive problems.

As always, the key is to listen to your body's feedback. Everyone's tolerance and digestive efficiency differ, and as a natural eater, you will gradually recognise what works best for you.

If you don't have regular access to creamy tropical fruits, a small amount of healthy fat can still support the absorption of fat-soluble vitamins such as A and E. Good sources include raw seeds, raw nuts, or naturally fatty fruits like avocado.

However, it's important to note that we are not heavy fat consumers, and most fruits naturally contain small amounts of fat. If you use any fatty ingredients, they should be consumed in moderation.

Highly Processed Food

Making sauce, dehydrating, hydrating, etc.

Some Raw food groups promote making *gourmet raw dishes* using various processes such as dehydration, hydration, mixing, and grinding. While these methods can make food more creative or convenient, it's important to understand *why* we eat and *how* to best support the body's natural processes.

Gourmet-style food may not always fulfil that purpose. During heavy processing, ingredients can become oxidised or nutrient-damaged, reducing their effectiveness and vitality. In addition, many components used in such recipes are not our body's natural foods and may irritate the digestive system.

As a general guideline, if you cannot make a meal from an ingredient on its own and enjoy it, it's best to minimise or avoid it. For example, you wouldn't eat a full plate of raw onion or garlic alone; the same principle applies to spices, chilli, salt, and pepper. These ingredients can have strong antibacterial properties that may disrupt the balance of beneficial bacteria in the intestines and interfere with gut flora.

Over-processing raw materials can undermine the very intention of a natural diet. When done regularly, it may even lead to similar imbalances experienced by those following the Typical Western Diet (T.W.D.), despite using raw ingredients.

Capture 12

Challenges

Any change in our life brings its challenges, and adopting a Natural Lifestyle with a Raw Vegan diet is no exception.

If you want to learn something new, you must dedicate time to study it. To benefit from your learning, you need to put that knowledge into practice and experience the outcome firsthand. Similarly, achieving Ultimate Health requires understanding what it truly means, taking consistent action, and then being amazed by the results.

Transitioning to a Raw lifestyle brings both changes and challenges. Here are a few I'd like to share.

Detox

The heavy detoxification (let's call it detox) process begins as soon as you stop introducing toxins into your body. This process is one of the main challenges of adopting a Raw Vegan lifestyle and often the reason many newcomers give up early.

When you start living naturally, your body begins detoxing almost immediately, sometimes even on the first day. To understand why, let's take a step back. When raw materials are heated during cooking, parts of the food can become toxic depending on the temperature and duration. Over time, these compounds accumulate in the body because our organs can only eliminate a certain amount of waste each day. The excess toxins are stored in our tissues and organs.

When we stop consuming cooked or processed food and begin eating naturally, the body finally gets the opportunity to **release stored toxins** into the bloodstream and remove them through natural detoxification pathways such as the liver, kidneys, lungs, and skin. This phase is sometimes referred to as *intensive detox*. I use this term because our bodies are always detoxing to some degree, regardless of diet, but when toxin intake drops, the body can focus on clearing older, stored waste.

As these toxins circulate through the bloodstream and lymphatic system, various organs may become temporarily stressed. This can trigger symptoms that resemble illness. The first two weeks of intensive detox are typically the most challenging. Many people experience temporary discomfort such as fatigue, flu-like symptoms, constipation, or diarrhoea.

These are not signs that your new lifestyle is harming you; they are often signs that your body is healing. The intensity and duration vary between individuals depending on factors such as prior diet, lifestyle, toxin load, and current health condition.

Some people experience **headaches**, while others notice **skin rashes** as the body pushes toxins out through the skin. You might also feel **dizzy, fatigued, sore,** or develop **pimples** or **nausea**. These reactions occur because the organs involved in detoxification are working hard to eliminate stored waste.

It's also common to feel **low in energy** as the detox process demands a lot from the body. Many people who are unaware of this natural adjustment period believe the Raw Vegan lifestyle "isn't for them" and quit too soon. I've seen this happen many times. Some people I encouraged to start the journey felt unwell in the first week and assumed something was wrong. They thought, *"I must need meat again!"* or *"My body can't handle this!"*

When they returned to their old eating habits, they felt temporary relief because reintroducing cooked and processed foods slowed the detox process and trapped toxins back in their tissues. This short-term "comfort" can be misleading and keeps people from progressing toward true healing.

A close friend once asked me, *"If Raw Veganism is so beneficial, why do people feel sick at first?"* The answer is simple: these symptoms aren't sickness; they're part of the healing process. Taking pain killers during this phase is not ideal and delays your body's natural recovery. That being said, detox symptoms can be eased or reduced by:

- Getting extra sleep and rest
- Drinking plenty of pure water
- Practising yoga or meditation
- Spending time in nature
- Doing light exercise

Incorporating these habits helps the body release toxins more smoothly. If you stay committed to your natural lifestyle and continue eating raw, living foods, your body will gradually cleanse itself, and your journey toward **Ultimate Health** will truly begin.

Depending on the level of accumulated toxins, detoxification can take months or even years, with varying intensity. However, the benefits of a **natural** lifestyle begin almost immediately; you'll notice small improvements in energy, clarity, and digestion from the first day.

During the first couple of weeks, it's normal to notice darker, stronger-smelling urine, this simply reflects toxins leaving your system. To support this process, I recommend drinking around 8–12 cups of pure, filtered water daily during this period. Hydration helps the body flush waste more effectively.

You may also experience **constipation**, especially early on. I encountered this in my second year of being fully Raw. It showed me how much waste had been stored in my body and how persistent some of it was! If this happens, eat one or two whole kiwifruits with the skin. Other natural laxative fruits, such as fresh figs or berries (special black berry), can also help. Gradually, your digestion will improve; one of the earliest signs that your body is regaining balance.

Light exercise can further accelerate detox. During activities like walking or gentle jogging, toxins are expelled through sweat, often producing an unpleasant odour. Over time, as your system purifies, your sweat becomes neutral. I noticed this transformation myself: years ago, I had to wash my sports clothes after every workout because of the smell. Now, after years of raw living, my sweat smells like clean water; proof that my body has thoroughly detoxed. You'll likely experience the same when your body reaches this state of purity.

Hot Food

Sometimes, people tell me how they can miss their hot foods, especially during a cold winter or when living in a cold climate. Let's think about hot food and how it is consumed.

When we cook food, we raise the temperature to at least 100 °C (212 °F). In some methods, such as deep frying, the temperature can reach 250 °C to 300 °C. So, we end up with really hot food, right? But can anyone eat food at 250 °C? Of course not, as it would burn our mouth and throat. What about food at 100 °C? Can we eat it immediately? Again, the answer is no. It would still burn us. So, what do we do? We let it cool down to a suitable temperature for our mouths. This temperature is usually between 30 °C and 40 °C, right?

Now you really do not eat hot food. Even if someone can handle the higher temperatures, say 60 or 70 °C (burning their mouth in the process, I know some people who do this!), once the food consumed, it quickly reaches thermal equilibrium with the body's internal temperature of around 37 °C. The sensation of heat from hot food is temporary and doesn't last long.

Some may still argue they feel the heat much longer when they have cooked food. let us discuss why people miss their hot food and how it is addressed after you continue the natural lifestyle path.

First, it is like any other addiction you might have had for years, and your body got used to it, similar to a smoker addicted to cigarettes. Transitioning to a natural path will bring health benefits to the body, and soon after, it won't crave hot food. It is like someone quitting smoking, and if they notice the health improvements, they may not want to go back.

Second, the unhealthy cells in the body crave hot food. When you switch to a Raw diet, these unhealthy cells usually die off due to the lack of their food. They are then replaced by healthy cells, and the craving for the unhealthy foods usually disappears.

The third and last one is when you consume raw food every day, your body generates a significant amount of energy, something it couldn't do with cooked and oxidised food. As a result, you don't need hot food to temporarily stimulate warmth. You feel the heat and energy within you all the time and won't crave that temporary sensation.

To discuss this in more detail, as I mentioned earlier in the book, the burning process of food in our body, known as metabolism, is the primary energy source for our activities. When we consume oxidised materials, such as cooked or highly processed food, our bodies cannot burn them again effectively. Consequently, energy production is compromised. How many people do you know who constantly feel cold and need to eat or drink something hot to feel warm for a short period? Keeping the body warm with hot food is only a mental effect and does not provide a sustained feeling of warmth.

When you eat proper raw food, it is ready to be metabolised efficiently, creating the necessary energy, and keeping you warm all the time. I feel real heat when I consume raw food. You may not imagine how much heat I feel in my stomach when I take a pear or two as my breakfast; I can feel the genuine burning sensation inside; You can test it yourself tomorrow morning and see how you feel.

When people eat heavily cooked or processed foods, toxic residues and excess fats can gradually clog blood vessels, particularly the small capillaries. These blocked pathways prevent red blood cells from efficiently delivering oxygen and nutrients to tissues. As a result, metabolism weakens and energy (and therefore body heat) declines.

Have you ever noticed how you feel the cold mostly in your fingertips, legs, and ears? That's because these areas have the smallest capillaries, which are the easiest to become obstructed by unhealthy fats and waste.

By transitioning to a proper Raw diet, the body begins to heal itself, dissolving stored fats and toxins and clearing the capillaries.

As they reopen, oxygen and nutrients flow freely again, allowing you to feel warmth, even in your hands and feet.

I personally experienced this transformation. Before going Raw, I had high blood pressure (around 140/90 mm Hg) and a resting heartbeat of 86 bpm. After just five weeks on a natural lifestyle, my blood pressure dropped to 100/60 mm Hg, and my pulse slowed to a healthy 60 bpm. These rapid improvements showed how efficiently my cardiovascular system recovered once the vessels were no longer burdened by toxins.

My wife often comments on how cold my hands feel to the touch, yet I don't feel cold inside. The surface skin may cool when exposed to air, but internally, my circulation keeps me comfortably warm.

Have you ever noticed feeling warm right after waking up on a cold morning? For those few minutes, before you start moving, you don't feel the chill. That's because during sleep we breathe more deeply, bringing in more oxygen and fuelling higher metabolism, which naturally generates heat.

When you follow a proper Raw lifestyle and complete the initial detox phase, your metabolism works at its best. You'll likely find that you feel warmer than most people on the Typical Western Diet (T.W.D.). Many raw eaters even reduce the number of clothing layers they need in winter and become less sensitive to cold overall.

Another helpful tip: after your daily shower, finish with a short burst of cold water. Start with just a few seconds and build up gradually. This simple practice as explained in another chapter, stimulates circulation, strengthens your immune system, and helps you stay warm long after leaving the bathroom.

In the first few weeks of transitioning to a natural lifestyle, if you still feel the need for hot food, you can gently warm your raw ingredients to about 40 to 45 °C, which is usually not damaging. This approach can help ease the transition until the initial detox processes subside, allowing you to experience the real energy within and gradually reduce cravings for hot food.

Teeth

I've often heard people say the reason we cook food is that cooked meals are softer and easier to digest. But can a cooked burger really be softer than a banana? That argument might make sense when comparing cooked food to hard-shelled nuts, but most fruits (except perhaps apples) are naturally soft and easy to eat.

Even if cooked food is easier to chew, the real issue may be that many people simply don't like chewing. Yet, chewing is an essential part of digestion. Even well-chewed cooked food remains harder to digest than raw food because heating alters its structure. Our bodies struggle with cooked food, it demands more enzymes and energy to break down and can even lead to constipation.

For those new to a Raw diet, hard fruits or soaked nuts may initially feel tough on the teeth, especially if there's existing damage caused by years of cooked and processed food, as was the case with mine. Remember, digestion begins in the mouth, not the stomach. Your teeth grind the food while your saliva enzymes begin converting carbohydrates into simple sugars that are absorbed into the bloodstream. That's why chewing slowly and thoroughly is critical. It gives your mouth time to perform its part of digestion before the food reaches the stomach.

People who eat quickly or talk while eating (especially when distracted by television or work) often fail to chew properly, which burdens the digestive system. In a natural lifestyle, most foods are fruits, which are generally soft enough to chew easily, even with sensitive teeth. The small portion of nuts should always be soaked for at least 24 hours to activate them and make them gentler on the teeth and stomach.

If necessary, you can use a grinder or food processor to help with chewing. However, minimise processed foods in your diet, once the protective layer of fruits, vegetables, or seeds is broken, oxidation begins quickly, reducing freshness and nutrient value. If you make processed food, eat it soon after preparation. You'll notice the colour darkening over time, a clear sign of oxidation and nutrient loss.

Sometimes, when transitioning to a Raw lifestyle, people notice an increase in tooth sensitivity or cavities. This usually stems from past enamel damage caused by cooked and processed foods combined with the natural fruit sugars now present in the diet. To prevent this, rinse your mouth with water after each meal. Simply swish a small amount of clean water in your mouth for a few seconds before swallowing or spitting it out.

Another excellent practice is oil pulling, ideally before bedtime after brushing. Swish a teaspoon of oil in your mouth for 3–5 minutes, then take it in or spit it out (without rinsing). Some practitioners prefer to do it before brushing, you can experiment and see what feels best. The best choice is vegan Omega-3 oil, which I personally use. I usually swish it around my mouth for a few minutes before swallowing, as it helps clean the gums and nourish the teeth. Other options include raw, cold-pressed, organic coconut oil, olive oil, flaxseed oil, or hemp seed oil. Make sure any oil you use is extra virgin and cold-pressed. With consistent practice, you'll likely notice fresher breath, stronger gums, and cleaner teeth within a few weeks.

A natural lifestyle provides the nutrients your teeth and bones need particularly calcium and Vitamin D, which work together to maintain strength and structure. Since adopting a Raw lifestyle, I've seen remarkable improvements in my oral health. My gums no longer bleed, my teeth feel stronger, and dental visits have become rare. I once believed bleeding gums were a normal result of flossing, now I know it was a sign of inflammation and imbalance. With time, patience, and proper nutrition, anyone embracing a Raw lifestyle can experience **similar improvements**.

Clothes

Besides all the other changes, one of the most noticeable yet enjoyable challenges when starting a natural lifestyle is your clothes!

By eating raw, living foods, your body naturally returns to its ideal weight. For most people, this means losing excess weight, while for others who are underweight, it can mean gaining healthy mass as the body rebuilds genuine cells and restores proper digestion.

When you consume natural foods, unhealthy cells die off and are eliminated, while new healthy cells regenerate to replace them. Over time, your body settles into its natural size and proportions. Because of this, you'll likely find that many (if not all) of your old clothes no longer fit.

For those carrying extra weight, the transformation often happens quickly. Stored fat and excess body water naturally reduce within 2 to 8 months, depending on your previous condition. Some people even reach their ideal weight within the first four weeks.

In my own experience, my waist size dropped from 34 to 28 inches, and I had to replace all my trousers. My shirt size changed from Large to Small/Extra Small, and I donated most of my wardrobe to charity including several brand-new suits I had never worn. Even my shoe size decreased slightly.

I understand that replacing so many clothes can feel like a challenge, but imagine this: you're at your ideal weight, full of energy, and eating real, delicious food every day. You wake up feeling lighter, healthier, and full of life, how amazing is that? When you look in the mirror and see yourself in your best physical shape, it becomes easy to care for your body and reward it with clothes that reflect your new vitality. *How wonderful will that feel?*

These days, I love spending more time treating my wonderfully healthy body with nice, brand-new clothes. I love myself much more than before, and I've noticed that other Raw Vegans I've met feel the same way. You'll almost certainly experience it too.

Dining and Travel

Once your body becomes cleaner and more balanced, you may notice that it reacts differently to certain foods you used to eat. Even small amounts of cooked or processed food can sometimes cause subtle changes in how you feel. In my early years of being fully Raw, I remember that even a small piece of bread would give me a headache, and a few bites of cooked vegetables could cause mild stomach discomfort or breakouts.

Over the years, I've noticed that my body has become more stable and less reactive. For example, on a recent seven-day cruise, where fresh raw options were limited, I ate small amounts of simple vegan low-heat cooked food and felt fine. My body handled it well, but as soon as I returned home, I naturally went back to my fully Raw lifestyle.

This experience reminded me that balance and awareness are key. The goal of living naturally is not perfection or restriction but understanding your body and choosing what truly supports it. Occasional exceptions while travelling or socialising do not undo the long-term benefits of a clean, natural lifestyle.

Social events, dining out, and travel can indeed be challenging, especially since many people are still unfamiliar with what a Raw lifestyle involves. When visiting friends or travelling, I often bring my own smoothies or choose simple, raw options such as salads made with leafy greens, lemon juice, and olive oil. When that's not possible, I look for the freshest fruits available and keep things flexible.

Fortunately, times are changing. Just as veganism has become mainstream, I believe Raw Vegan options will soon follow. With the rapid spread of information, we're already seeing encouraging signs. Some airlines, including Emirates (when I travelled with them a couple of years ago), offered Raw Vegan meals, and many restaurants, especially in the USA, have begun including Raw Vegan items or even entire menus.

Of course, there will still be moments when it's not easy to find what you want. But with preparation, understanding, and a positive mindset, you can navigate these situations gracefully. Over time, your vibrant energy and health will speak for themselves, inspiring others to explore this way of living. As more people embrace natural, unprocessed food, dining out, social gatherings, and travel will become even easier and more enjoyable for everyone.

From my experience, the first 6 to 12 months of being fully Raw are the most important for cleansing the body. During this phase, the body focuses on eliminating long-accumulated toxins and restoring natural balance. Once this deep cleansing stage is complete, the body's detoxification system becomes stronger and more resilient, able to handle small amounts of simple cooked vegan food without the same strong reactions as before. While cooked food is still not ideal compared to being fully raw, having a small portion occasionally, especially in social settings or while travelling can be acceptable. It allows flexibility without compromising your long-term health journey or the benefits gained through a Raw lifestyle.

Your Senses

The final challenge in adopting a natural lifestyle lies within your senses. As your body clears toxins, your organs begin to function more efficiently, especially those involved in sensory perception. You gradually return to a natural state of living, where every part of your body including your eyes, ears, tongue, and nose operates at its best. Over time, these organs often lose sensitivity due to toxins introduced mainly through cooked and processed foods.

With a clean, natural lifestyle, everything changes. Many people who transition to this way of living notice significant improvements in eyesight, with some even reducing or no longer needing glasses. Interestingly, a few have reported their eye colour becoming lighter or returning to its original shade after years on a Raw Vegan lifestyle. The eyes are highly responsive organs, often reflecting the body's internal health. As they clear of toxins, they can become clearer, brighter, and more radiant, contributing to a natural, healthy glow that enhances the beauty of your face.

When your body is nourished with living foods, your senses return to their natural sharpness. You begin to truly taste your food, its real sweetness, freshness, and vitality. Smells become more distinct, and eating turns into an entirely new experience of appreciation and connection.

However, heightened senses can also present new challenges. Once your sense of smell becomes more refined, strong artificial or unpleasant odours, such as cigarette smoke, perfumes, or the smell of some food can become overwhelming. Crowded places or fish markets, for example, might feel unpleasant at first. It's important to understand that unpleasant body odours are often a sign of internal toxicity. When the body is overloaded with waste, it attempts to release these toxins through sweat and breath, which is why products like perfumes, deodorants, mouth sprays, and gums are so common. These, however, only mask the problem temporarily rather than addressing the cause.

For those living a natural lifestyle, this can be a noticeable challenge, especially at the beginning. A simple and pleasant solution is to use natural, cold-pressed essential oils on the body or clothes before social events, or to wear a light mask when needed. Over time, you'll likely become more comfortable and less reactive as your body and its senses continue to adjust.

As more people embrace a cleaner, natural lifestyle, we can look forward to a fresher, healthier world, one where both our bodies and our environment carry the **purity of natural living**.

Capture 13

Other Requirements for Your Ultimate Health

While we have discussed the importance of maintaining an appropriate diet and selecting the right foods, it's essential to recognise that other crucial aspects of our lives also require attention to attain optimal health and happiness. In the following list, we will explore each of these aspects individually and understand their significance.

Enough Deep Sleep

Sleep is one of the most vital yet often overlooked pillars of health. Everyone needs proper rest each night to restore both mind and body. As discussed earlier in the section on circadian rhythm, the third cycle, beginning around 8 p.m. and ending around 4 a.m., is the most beneficial window for deep rest and repair. During this time, the body focuses on recovery, nutrient absorption, and cellular maintenance. Sleeping during this period allows the body and mind to rejuvenate fully and ensures the absorption system operates at its best.

Unfortunately, many people continue eating or stimulating themselves during these hours, which can interfere with digestion and leave them feeling sluggish the next morning. Have you ever noticed feeling heavy or tired after a late-night meal?

When we sleep, our bodies shift from a **catabolic state** to an **anabolic state**. In the catabolic phase (daytime), the body burns food materials to generate energy for physical and mental activities. In the anabolic phase (during sleep), it conserves energy for repair, detoxification, and tissue rebuilding.

Our internal 24-hour clock (the **circadian rhythm**) remains consistent no matter what time you go to bed or wake up. This rhythm controls hormone release, regulating energy, mood, and sleep. For example, **melatonin**, the hormone responsible for sleep, is secreted by the pineal gland after about 8 p.m. when darkness falls. Its levels peak between 1 a.m. and 2 a.m., then gradually decline by 4 a.m. to 8 a.m. Exposure to light (even small amounts) can suppress melatonin production and disrupt sleep. Therefore, sleeping in total darkness is essential, avoid leaving on lamps, screens, or "night lights," regardless of colour.

In contrast, the hormone **cortisol** rises with morning light, signalling the body to wake up. This natural rise in cortisol prepares us to be alert and active for the day ahead. Proper deep sleep is crucial not only for physical restoration but also for brain repair, in fact, certain genes are only activated in the brain during deep sleep.

While body detoxification mainly occurs through the lymphatic system, the brain has no lymph nodes or vessels. Instead, it relies on a specialised waste-clearance system called the **glymphatic system**. This system circulates cerebrospinal fluid (CSF) through the brain's tissues to flush out waste products like beta-amyloid and tau proteins substances linked to neurodegenerative diseases such as Alzheimer's. The glymphatic system is most active during deep sleep, when brain cells temporarily shrink to allow more efficient fluid exchange. This is one of the key reasons deep, uninterrupted sleep is vital and why lack of it may lead to headaches or brain fog upon waking.

Determining how much sleep you need, and improving its quality, (especially deep sleep) is essential for maintaining optimal health. While it's often suggested that most people require around eight hours of sleep each night, this varies depending on individual factors and lifestyle. Starting with eight hours as a general guide is reasonable, but with a proper natural lifestyle, many find they naturally need less, while others may still require more.

Listening to your body is key. If you can wake up without an alarm and feel fully refreshed, it's a good sign that you've had enough deep, restorative sleep.

Several factors can affect sleep quality, including eating late at night, noise, exposure to light in the bedroom, high stress levels, medications, and major life changes. People such as airline crew, shift workers, or parents with newborns often find it especially challenging to get proper sleep due to demanding schedules. Regardless of circumstances, it's important to create an environment that mimics natural living as closely as possible and to prioritise rest as a foundation for good health.

Try to maintain a consistent bedtime every night even on weekends and keep your sleep environment calm and comfortable. Adjust room temperature to suit your needs, using a blanket or gentle air conditioning if necessary. Minimise screen use before bed and avoid stimulating content such as news or social media, which can disturb your mind and delay sleep. In fact, limiting exposure to daily news altogether can often improve both mental clarity and sleep quality, as much of it tends to focus on negative or stressful events.

Be mindful of substances that interfere with deep rest. Cooked meals eaten late, alcohol, coffee, tea, smoking, and even some supplements can all affect sleep quality. For example, iodine tablets are best taken in the morning, as they can sometimes interfere with sleep when consumed at night. Alcohol in particular can disrupt deep sleep cycles, leading to restlessness and reduced mood the following day, a pattern many people notice after weekends of social drinking.

With a proper natural lifestyle and a supportive environment, deep and refreshing sleep often becomes effortless. You'll wake up feeling clear, energised, and ready for the day, and yes even on **Monday mornings**!

Mental Health

You've probably heard that our physical and mental health are deeply connected; and they truly are. A relaxed body supports a calm, balanced mind, while ongoing stress can directly affect physical functions. The digestive system, for example, is highly sensitive to stress and often struggles to perform efficiently under tension, which can hinder nutrient absorption. At the same time, deficiencies in nutrients such as the B-vitamin group and zinc can impair nerve function and worsen stress levels, creating a cycle of anxiety, fatigue, and poor health.

Have you ever felt anxious for no clear reason? This often happens when the body is under hidden stress, even when we're not consciously aware of it.

When we face a stressful situation, the body naturally releases hormones (mainly **adrenaline** and **cortisol**) to help us respond to the challenge. This instinctive "fight or flight" reaction evolved to protect us from immediate danger. Thousands of years ago, if a person walking through the forest suddenly encountered a wild animal, their body would release these stress hormones to heighten alertness, increase heart rate, and redirect blood flow to the muscles, preparing them to act quickly. During this time, other functions, such as digestion and immunity are temporarily reduced, as the body prioritises survival. Once the threat passes, the body gradually metabolises and clears cortisol and adrenaline through the liver, kidneys, and lymphatic system, allowing it to return to balance.

This system works perfectly for short-term stress, but in modern life, most stressors are mental, emotional, or social, work pressure, financial worries, relationships, and constant digital stimulation. When stress hormones stay elevated for too long, the body struggles to return to repair mode, leading to fatigue, digestive issues, inflammation, and eventually more serious health problems.

People who follow the Typical Western Diet (T.W.D.) are often more prone to chronic stress, partly due to poor nutrition and the overconsumption of processed foods. The brain and nervous system rely on nutrients such as omega-3 fatty acids, magnesium, zinc, and B-vitamins to regulate mood and manage stress. When these are missing or poorly absorbed, emotional balance becomes harder to maintain, leading to irritability and tension.

Chronic stress also affects digestion. When cortisol remains elevated, blood flow to the digestive tract decreases, reducing enzyme activity and slowing bowel movements. Over time, this can cause constipation, which further disrupts gut health and nutrient absorption, creating a feedback loop between stress and digestion.

Prolonged stress has wider effects on the body. High cortisol levels suppress the immune system and promote inflammation, contributing to fatigue and vulnerability to infection. Research (see References) suggests chronic stress plays a role in many diseases, from autoimmune and cardiovascular conditions to metabolic and mental health disorders.

So, how can we manage chronic stress? The first step is adopting a natural lifestyle. When the body receives clean, raw nutrition and functions efficiently, stress levels tend to decrease naturally. It's rare for someone on a consistent Raw diet to experience ongoing stress in the same way as those consuming cooked or processed foods.

Of course, stressful events still happen, through work, family, or life circumstances. But when your organs function well and your digestive system is clean, your body can process stress hormones quickly and return to equilibrium. As you become healthier and more in tune with your body, you'll start recognising subtle internal signals that help you restore calm before stress builds up.

A natural lifestyle also enhances the detoxification systems; the liver, kidneys, lymphatic flow, and even breathing which help remove excess cortisol and other stress metabolites. This is one reason why people who eat raw, whole foods often experience greater resilience, clarity, and emotional stability.

A balanced diet, deep restorative sleep, regular exercise, and conscious breathing form the foundation of mental and emotional health. While we've already discussed food and sleep, exercise and breathing will be covered later in this chapter.

If you're still transitioning away from unhealthy foods, these small, practical steps can already help reduce daily stress:

- Stay hydrated with pure, clean water, as outlined in the hydration chapter.

- Eat slowly in a quiet, relaxed environment without distractions like television or mobile phones.

- Take short daily walks to stimulate circulation and clear the mind.

- Practice meditation or gentle yoga for a few minutes each day; even simple breath awareness helps.

- Establish a consistent bedtime routine, ideally around 10:00 p.m. to align with your body's natural rhythm.

- Switch off electronic devices before sleep and rest in a dark, quiet room to encourage deep, restorative rest.

Exercise

Oh, exercising; what a wonderful word! How often have you heard that daily exercise is crucial for your health? What kind of picture comes to mind when you hear the word "exercise"? A man or woman covered in sweat with a sports bottle in their hand? Or perhaps someone running outdoors or lifting weights in a gym?

Some people feel intimidated by images of heavy workouts or exhausted athletes, but exercise doesn't need to be extreme. Let's set aside those pictures for a moment and explore why movement is so important, and how you can make it part of your daily routine in a way that truly supports your health.

I remember years ago when I started going to the gym almost every day. I asked one of my close friends to join me, and his response was, "Sports and exercising are not good for my smoking!" He was absolutely right, because it's hard to continue smoking once you start exercising regularly. Toxins like nicotine make physical performance much harder, while exercise naturally encourages the body to reject such toxins.

We all move to some degree each day, walking, standing, or doing chores. Even people confined to bed still make small movements, as the body cannot function without them. But human life was not always so sedentary. In earlier times, people spent much of their day outdoors, walking, running, climbing, or working physically. Even just a century ago, daily life required far more movement than it does today.

Modern conveniences, cars, machinery, and technology have made life easier but also far less active. Sitting in cars, at desks, or in front of screens for most of the day limits the natural movement our bodies rely on. That's why daily, intentional exercise is now essential for maintaining health.

The **lymphatic system** is one of the key reasons why. Unlike the cardiovascular system, the lymphatic system has no pump, it relies on **body movement** to circulate lymph fluid and remove cellular waste. Regular movement helps flush toxins through the body so they can be expelled via the liver, kidneys, and skin.

Exercise also boosts **metabolism**, supports oxygen delivery, and strengthens the heart, muscles, and bones. It helps burn food efficiently, improves digestion, and increases energy. Another great benefit is mental calmness, exercise releases **endorphins**, the "feel-good" hormones that reduce stress and promote emotional balance.

It's generally recommended to engage in at least **30 minutes of activity per day**, enough to raise your heart rate slightly and work up a gentle sweat. It doesn't have to be intense; even a brisk walk, dancing, or cycling can be highly beneficial. The key is to move more than your normal daily routine.

We've already talked about how movement supports lymph flow, but **vertical movement** (up-and-down motion) is especially important. Research (see References) suggests that this type of movement helps stimulate lymphatic circulation throughout the whole body and can even improve **bone density**, reducing the risk of osteoporosis when combined with a proper natural lifestyle.

One of the best vertical exercises is **jumping on a trampoline** (a rebounder). It's small, fun, and effective. A gym trampoline about one metre wide and forty centimetres tall, it fits easily at home or in the office. Jumping around 300 times a day even in short sessions can make a big difference. I keep one in my office and jump for a few minutes whenever I've been sitting too long.

Now, let's talk about something that's not often mentioned; **breast movement and health**. I've come across studies and statistics highlighting the rising number of breast cancer cases in women today. According to Australian government statistics, in Australia about **57 women** are diagnosed with breast cancer **every day**, which adds up to over 20,000 new cases each year, and sadly, around **nine** lives are **lost** daily to this disease.

While many factors contribute to breast cancer, poor diet and toxin accumulation in soft tissues may play a role. The breasts, being composed largely of fatty tissue, can accumulate these substances over time. Limited movement and restricted circulation in the chest area especially from wearing tight bras may reduce lymphatic drainage, allowing toxins to linger longer than they should.

Sports bras, while providing support, often limit breast movement even further. This might unintentionally reduce the natural lymphatic flow that helps the body cleanse itself. Allowing freer movement during certain exercises, even if initially uncomfortable, can support better circulation and overall breast health.

Ultimately, **no movement means limited lymph flow**, and over time, that can compromise detoxification. Prioritising health over temporary comfort is worthwhile and incorporating more natural movement can be a valuable part of long-term wellbeing.

Running, jogging, or rebounding are all excellent forms of vertical movement. Mix it up, jump high, low, twist, use single-leg and double-leg motions to engage different muscle groups and maximise the benefits. Make movement a daily habit: it's convenient, energising, and one of the most enjoyable ways to care for your body.

Before engaging in activities such as jumping on a trampoline, daily exercise, or taking cold showers or plunges, it's essential to discuss them with your healthcare professional and obtain their approval. This is particularly crucial if you have any underlying health issues or chronic diseases such as cardiovascular diseases, diabetes, or arthritis.

Cold Shower

A cold shower or cold plunge is another excellent activity that can help you reach your Ultimate Health. Once again, this connects closely to the **lymphatic system** and body movement. When cold water touches your skin, it causes the surface tissues and internal organs to contract. This rhythmic contraction helps stimulate lymph flow, supporting detoxification throughout the body.

You may have heard that professional athletes use cold-water immersion after intense exercise or competition. During vigorous activity, the body produces **lactic acid**, which needs to be cleared efficiently by the lymphatic system for recovery and continued performance. A cold shower or ice bath helps accelerate this process by reducing inflammation, flushing out metabolic waste, and restoring balance. For athletes, this "cold therapy" is an essential part of recovery.

Even for non-athletes, cold exposure offers powerful benefits. A daily cold shower can strengthen the **immune system**, enhance circulation, and improve resistance to illness. Alternating between hot and cold water (sometimes called **contrast therapy**) creates expansion and contraction in blood vessels and tissues, acting almost like an internal massage. This gentle "massage" helps the lymphatic system function more effectively, supporting detoxification and overall vitality.

Taking a cold shower after exercise or at the end of your regular shower routine is a great practice. Two to three minutes is enough. If the water feels too cold in winter, start with just a few seconds and gradually increase over time. Alternatively, immersing yourself in a **cold plunge bath** can offer the same benefits; though not everyone has access to one.

In warmer climates, where tap water may not be very cold, you can enhance the experience by adding **ice** to your bath or using a **portable cold plunge tub**. The contrast between hot and cold temperatures benefits the lymphatic system and mimics a deep tissue massage involving nearly all internal organs. The sense of refreshment and calm that follows a cold shower or plunge is truly remarkable.

Deep Breathing

So far, we've discussed food, proper diet, and other essentials for robust health; including the importance of drinking pure water. But what about **air** and the clean oxygen our bodies need for Ultimate Health?

We can survive days without food and water, but only a few minutes without oxygen. This shows how vital breathing is. Through breathing, the body removes **carbon dioxide** and airborne impurities from the lungs, while deep breathing increases oxygen levels in the blood, supporting key detox organs such as the liver and kidneys.

Breathing is not only a physical act; it's also deeply connected to our **mental and emotional state**. Our breathing patterns often mirror how we feel, shallow and quick when we're stressed or angry, deep and steady when we're calm or in nature. Conversely, when we consciously slow and deepen our breath, we can calm the mind, even in tense situations.

The mind and body are strongly interconnected. A relaxed body supports a peaceful mind, and a calm mind allows the body to function efficiently. It's difficult for a sick person to feel happy, whereas someone in good health can more easily return to a balanced emotional state. Diaphragmatic breathing(or deep breathing) plays an important role in achieving this harmony.

Deep breathing has been widely studied and written[1] about, so I won't go into great technical detail here. You can explore different methods and find what feels best for you. But in essence, it's not

---

[1] Breath, The New Science of a Lost Art- Book by James Nestor is a good one to read.

complicated. The goal is to **breathe deeply into your abdomen**, allowing your diaphragm to expand. This brings more oxygen into your lungs and bloodstream.

Interestingly, this is how we naturally breathe during sleep, and how children breathe in their early years, before they're taught to hold their breath or suppress emotions through shallow breathing.

Deep breathing activates the **parasympathetic nervous system**, which promotes relaxation, steadies the heart rate, and supports digestion. When the body is calm, nutrient absorption and overall function improve.

In addition to breathing deeply, it's equally important to ensure **access to clean, fresh air** every day. Open your windows regularly, even in winter to let oxygen circulate through your home. If your air conditioning system doesn't supply fresh air, indoor plants can help by converting CO_2 into oxygen, improving air quality.

If you live in an area with polluted air, consider using an **air filtration system** at home. Also, try to avoid intense exercise outdoors during times of poor air quality, especially early in the morning or on cold, foggy days when pollution tends to linger.

Keep practicing your deep breathing daily, even for just a few minutes at a time. You'll soon notice its remarkable effects, greater calm, clearer focus, and a more energised body and mind.

Fasting

You've likely heard about fasting and its positive effects on health. Our body constantly detoxifies itself, but this process is limited by the capacity of its detox organs. When we stop eating, we give these organs more energy and time to focus on cleansing; that's the power of fasting. The energy usually used for digestion is redirected toward detoxification, allowing the body to eliminate waste more efficiently and restore balance.

Let's look more closely at fasting, as it's an important topic for anyone following a natural lifestyle.

Before starting, it's important to note that if you've been a Raw eater for some time, your body may already have a high detox capacity. In this case, fasting may only be needed occasionally or for short periods. In some cases, it might not be necessary at all. Fasting isn't suitable for everyone, regardless of diet or lifestyle. If your nutritional reserves are already at an optimal level, there might not be enough stored energy to support essential functions during fasting.

I emphasise this because some Raw Vegan educators promote fasting as something that should be done regularly; but excessive fasting can be risky. It can lead to malnutrition or, in extreme cases, cause irreversible organ damage.

As a committed Raw Vegan, especially if you eat mostly organic fruits, your body already functions at a high level of efficiency. Occasional fasting when done thoughtfully and with clear purpose may be beneficial, but it should never be overdone.

Types of Fasting

Fasting generally means avoiding certain types of food or drink for a specific period. I categorise fasting into four main types:

- **Dry fasting**

- **Juice fasting**

- **Mono-fruit fasting**

- **Water fasting**

There are also other variations, such as fasting until 4 p.m., intermittent fasting, or temporary vegan fasting (avoiding animal products for a period). These can all have their own effects, but here, we'll focus on the four main types. Each has unique benefits and potential risks, which we'll explore in the following sections.

Dry fasting

As the name suggests, dry fasting means not consuming any food or drink at all. This type of fasting mostly recommended in some religions and philosophies and is usually practiced for a short period, such as during daylight hours from sunrise to sunset. During this fasting method, individuals consume food and beverages at night, specifically between sunset and sunrise.

Dry fasting can have health benefits related to detoxification or autophagy[1]. However, it is primarily intended to enhance human

---

[1] **Autophagy** (from Greek, meaning "self-eating") is the body's natural process of cleaning out damaged or unnecessary cells. (see Glossary)

belief, determination, and compassion for those in poverty who lack access to food and water.

In terms of health, dry fasting may offer a short period of detoxification, although in a limited capacity since the organs involved in detoxification require water, which is avoided during dry fasting.

However, the energy saved by halting digestion can aid in detoxification. Some people practice dry fasting for extended periods, such as a few days, which can be dangerous. We cannot live without water for long, and prolonged dry fasting can cause irreversible damage to organs like the kidneys and liver.

Dry fasting isn't advisable for health as its benefits are limited and may even be nonexistent, especially if someone overeats at night when our digestive system should be resting, as discussed in the "When to Eat" chapter. Unless required for a religious ceremony and done only during the daytime, dry fasting should be avoided as a regular practice.

Juice fasting

Juice fasting has become increasingly popular and is often promoted as a quick way to lose weight or "detox." Many people find it appealing because fruit juice contains natural sugars that help reduce hunger and provide an immediate sense of energy. Juice fasts can range from a few days to several weeks, with some individuals reporting notable benefits such as improved energy and lighter digestion.

One reason juice fasting may feel effective is that it requires little energy for digestion, allowing the body to redirect resources toward detoxification. This can temporarily enhance the feeling of vitality and lightness.

However, I generally do not recommend juice fasting, especially when the juices are made primarily from sweet fruits and consumed in large quantities throughout the day. Without the natural fibre present in whole fruits, juices can place extra pressure on the pancreas by triggering a rapid insulin response to manage the sudden increase in blood sugar.

Moreover, when fibre is removed, the digestion of juice becomes too quick (much like drinking water) which reduces the time available for nutrient absorption. As a result, the body may not fully benefit from the vitamins and minerals present in the fruits or vegetables.

That said, certain forms of juice fasting, particularly those using mostly **low-sugar vegetable juices** with some fibre retained can be more balanced and less stressful on the body. They may provide a mild detox effect while maintaining better blood sugar stability and digestive comfort.

Mono fruit fasting

As the name suggests, mono-fruit fasting means eating only one type of fruit for a set period. This method can offer several benefits, such as increased energy, improved digestion, reduced inflammation, and enhanced detoxification. Many people also report clearer skin, weight loss, and faster recovery from certain health conditions.

Mono-fruit fasting can be a helpful way to transition into a Raw Fruitarian (Raw Vegan) lifestyle, especially for those who are significantly overweight, dealing with complex health issues, or not yet ready for water fasting. Because fruit naturally satisfies hunger, it makes this type of fast easier to maintain while still supporting cleansing and healing.

When done properly and with understanding of the body's needs, mono-fruit fasting can bring many benefits. However, it's important to remember that not all fruits are suitable for this approach. The chosen fruit should be juicy and hydrating enough to assist detoxification. For example, bananas are not ideal due to their low water content, whereas oranges, grapes, and melons are excellent options because they contain a balanced mix of natural sugars, water, and fibre.

I've personally tested all three, and they work well when done correctly. Some individuals have taken this further for instance, **Dr. Robert Morse** described in *The Detox Miracle Sourcebook* his experience of a year-long mono-orange fast using high-quality fruit, while **Anne Osborne** shared that she fasted on melons for six months and found it deeply transformative.

That said, these examples are not recommendations for long-term fasting. Such extended practices were more likely undertaken as personal experiments to observe bodily responses. In most cases, prolonged mono-fasting is unnecessary.

As always, listen closely to your body. When you live naturally, your body communicates clearly signalling when to eat, when to fast, and when to stop. With experience, proper research, and guidance from qualified practitioners, you'll learn what works best for you without resorting to extremes.

Water fasting

Water fasting involves abstaining from all food and consuming only water for a set period. The duration can range from 24 hours to several days, depending on individual goals and health conditions. Some people with serious health issues have reportedly fasted for extended periods (even up to 6 or 8 weeks) but always under the close supervision of an experienced fasting practitioner.

The water used should be pure, free from toxins and chemicals. Many educators recommend filtered or distilled water, as it contains minimal impurities. During a fast, it's best to drink according to thirst, not excessively, since overhydration can also place stress on the body. In my own experience, I tend to drink about the same amount as I normally would.

When done correctly and for the right reasons, water fasting can offer profound benefits. It allows the body to rest, repair, and eliminate damaged or unhealthy cells while stimulating the regeneration of new ones. Some people have reported recovery or significant improvement in conditions such as arthritis, asthma, autoimmune disorders, and cardiovascular issues through properly guided water fasting.

The duration of fasting depends on several factors, including the individual's health status, physical strength, and the nature of the condition being addressed. In some cases, long-term water fasting (up to 60 days) has been undertaken successfully under medical supervision. However, such extended fasts are **not suitable or safe for everyone**, and supervision by a qualified expert is essential.

It's also important to note that advanced or chronic diseases may not be fully reversible. In these situations, water fasting might not offer a complete cure, but it can still provide significant relief, improved energy, and a deep sense of clarity and renewal.

The detoxification process reaches its **peak efficiency** during water fasting, as all digestive activity stops and the body can redirect its full energy toward healing. For many, the mental clarity and lightness that follow are among the most rewarding experiences of all.

Which type of fasting is the best?

From health point of view the main purpose of all fasting methods, whether dry, juice, mono-fruit, or water is detoxification. This occurs on two levels: **physical**, by allowing the body to eliminate toxins and rest its digestive system, and **mental**, by strengthening determination, focus, and compassion.

From the four main fasting types discussed earlier, I've found that water fasting is the most effective for short periods, while mono-fruit fasting works well for longer durations, depending on individual needs and conditions.

I generally do not recommend juice fasting, as the health benefits it offers are not superior to those of other fasting methods or to those gained from following a proper natural Raw lifestyle.

Dry fasting, on the other hand, should be approached with caution. It may be acceptable for short, religious purposes but is not recommended for health reasons. Water is essential for detoxification, and extended dry fasting can damage the kidneys, liver, or other organs. Some educators suggest practicing short nightly dry fasts (mainly from sunset to sunrise) but this period coincides naturally with sleep, when we typically refrain from eating or drinking anyway.

Among all types, **water fasting** remains the best for **rapid detoxification**. Because the digestive system requires almost no energy, the body can direct its full energy toward cleansing, repair, and rejuvenation. Water fasting can also help initiate healing in individuals with chronic conditions such as autoimmune diseases or certain cancers. It is especially beneficial for those who have followed the Typical Western Diet (T.W.D.) for years and wish to transition toward a cleaner, natural lifestyle. Water fasting helps eliminate toxins and unhealthy cells quickly, often bringing back energy and mental clarity, giving people the motivation they need to continue their journey toward Ultimate Health.

Should you practice fasting?

When you maintain a natural lifestyle with a healthy Raw diet, you may only need to fast occasionally, and often for short periods, or not at all. Pure Raw eaters usually have limited storage of fat, glycogen, calcium, and vitamin B12. During fasting, when food intake stops, the body draws on these reserves to sustain essential functions until they're depleted.

In a healthy lifestyle, the body's detoxification capacity generally matches the level of toxins present. Nutrient stores are also balanced, so there's little excess that needs to be burned during fasting. Regular intake of fresh, raw foods ensures the body receives a continuous supply of nutrients, eliminating the need to store large reserves.

However, at times, your body may signal a need for rest; and fasting can be part of that process. As mentioned earlier, the body communicates through signals, but many people fail to recognise them, being distracted by pain, illness, medication, or daily stress. When living naturally and eating raw foods, your system becomes more sensitive and balanced, allowing you to interpret these signals clearly. You'll intuitively know when to fast, and when it's time to eat again.

In general, only short fasts are needed when following a proper natural lifestyle. If you ever feel the need for a longer fast, it should be done under the guidance of a professional fasting expert.

Personally, I fast occasionally, usually stopping when my body tells me to which often happens after three or four days. When I end a water fast, I transition with a mono-fruit fast for a day or two before returning to my regular Raw diet, as described in the "My Feast" chapter.

It's worth mentioning that **overeating** is a common issue for everyone, whether they follow the Typical Western Diet (T.W.D.) or a natural Raw diet. Overeating places unnecessary strain on the digestive system and can hinder nutrient absorption. Some people tend to overeat after fasting, believing they need to "make up" for nutrients lost, but this can cancel out many of the fasting benefits.

Fasting also brings a heightened **awareness of food and eating habits**. When you finish a water fast and take your first bite of solid fruit, the sensation is extraordinary, full of life, sweetness, and appreciation. It's an experience that words can hardly describe; you simply have to feel it yourself.

Beyond the physical benefits, fasting fosters gratitude. It helps you understand the true value of food and reminds you how often we eat mindlessly, rushing through meals to return to work or distractions. After fasting, each bite feels sacred. You eat slowly, consciously, and with deep appreciation for the nourishment nature provides.

Note: **Autophagy and Scientific Evidence**

Water fasting may stimulate a process called *autophagy*, the body's natural mechanism for breaking down and recycling old or damaged cells. This process is believed to support cellular repair, longevity, and overall detoxification.

However, while early research and anecdotal evidence suggest promising results, scientific understanding of autophagy in humans, particularly during fasting, is still evolving. Similarly, claims about fasting curing or reversing diseases such as cancer or autoimmune disorders are not yet supported by mainstream medical consensus.

That said, many studies recognise that properly supervised fasting can improve metabolic health, inflammation, and general wellbeing. As always, fasting should be approached with mindfulness and, when done for extended periods or medical reasons, under professional supervision.

Capture 14

Returns

I am confident that, in the near future, more people will embrace a natural lifestyle and experience the incredible benefits of a Raw Vegan diet.

As someone who has lived this lifestyle and seen its results firsthand, I encourage everyone to experience being fully Raw for a period of time. The changes that occur when the body receives only clean, living foods are remarkable and the benefits begin from the very first day you stop introducing processed or unhealthy substances into your system.

To reach a stable and balanced state of health, I recommend maintaining a 100% Raw Vegan lifestyle for at least 6 to 12 months, depending on your current diet, body condition, and level of commitment. After this period, you'll be in an excellent position to decide whether this way of living suits you long term.

Some people in the natural health community choose to be partially Raw, for example, 70% or 80% Raw; or follow the "Raw until 4 p.m." approach, where cooked vegan food is eaten in the evening. This can offer genuine benefits, especially during the transition phase, helping the body adapt gradually. However, partial Raw diets may slow the full detoxification process compared to being completely Raw. During the day, as the body processes fresh, raw foods, it begins releasing stored metabolic by-products and other waste materials. Returning to cooked or heavily processed foods later can interrupt this process and make progress less noticeable. Still, a gradual transition remains valuable; it's often the most practical and sustainable way to change habits without overwhelming the body or mind.

Some people prefer to move step by step, progressing from the Typical Western Diet (T.W.D.) to vegetarian, then vegan, and finally to Raw Vegan. Others transition more directly, depending on their health, lifestyle, and determination. Both paths can work effectively; the key is consistency and self-awareness.

In the early stages, you may experience **frequent hunger**. This is not a sign of deficiency but rather an adaptation period. Raw foods are lighter than cooked foods and digest faster, so you may feel hungry more often until your body adjusts. Over time, as your digestion becomes more efficient and your metabolism balances, these sensations typically subside.

When transitioning, it's also important to understand that your gut microbiome(the community of bacteria in your digestive system) adapts to your new diet. The microbes that thrive on cooked or processed foods begin to decrease, while those that digest raw plant foods become dominant. This change can temporarily influence cravings and mood, but it's a healthy part of rebalancing.

With patience and consistency, your body learns to thrive on raw foods, and you begin to feel lighter, clearer, and more energised; a reflection of the harmony between your internal environment and nature.

It's common for people to return to old habits when they misinterpret the body's adjustment signals. After switching to raw foods, many feel an empty stomach more often and mistake it for hunger. They may believe their body "needs" cooked food, when in reality, it's simply adapting to a lighter, faster-digesting diet. The familiarity of feeling "full" can be comforting, so they return to eating the way they did on the Typical Western Diet (T.W.D.).

For some, the intensity of early detox symptoms also makes them doubt the process and seek relief in cooked or processed foods.

How can you stay consistent through these challenges? The answer lies in **knowledge** and **determination**. Understanding what happens inside the body and why makes it easier to stay committed. When you learn how processed food affects digestion, hormones, and the nervous system, it becomes clearer why returning to it can delay progress.

Determination, however, is what carries you through. I once knew a woman who had been Raw Vegan for six years and she was a **professional chef** working with cooked food every day. Yet she never tried any of her dishes. The hardest part for her was seasoning her meals without sampling them. But her perseverance paid off. She mentioned that one of her greatest joys was being mistaken for her daughter's sister; a powerful reminder of how visibly the body responds to a clean lifestyle.

As your digestive system adjusts to natural, raw foods, your sensations also refine. The feeling of hunger becomes more accurate. Personally, I love the feeling of lightness that comes with this lifestyle; being active, clear-minded, and full of energy. It's astonishing how something as simple as one or two pears can feel like a complete breakfast. Years ago, my breakfast table was heavy with bread, butter, cheese, eggs, honey and jam; all of which left me sluggish and bloated. I used to reach for tea or coffee to numb the discomfort. Now, with raw foods, my mornings are easy, energising, and pain-free.

When the body is burdened by processed or heavy foods, nerve signalling can become less efficient due to inflammation, poor circulation, and metabolic imbalance. Once you cleanse and nourish your body naturally, these communication pathways improve, you begin to recognise your body's subtle messages more clearly and respond appropriately.

Embracing a natural lifestyle allows you to reconnect with all your senses (strong and pleasant) and makes it easier to perceive the genuine signals from your body. Your body is constantly communicating with you, indicating whether your actions are right or wrong. As you continue with this natural lifestyle, these signals become clearer, and you'll become more attuned to even the subtlest messages.

As your body becomes cleaner and more efficient, it may also become more sensitive to certain foods. When you reintroduce highly processed or heavy animal-based foods after being Raw Vegan for a while, your body can react strongly; not because it's "weaker," but because it has become more finely tuned.

To me even a small piece of bread can sometimes give me a headache. Years ago, I considered wholemeal bread one of the healthiest foods in my pantry. I never imagined I'd reach a level of wellbeing where bread would feel heavy and unpleasant.

It's interesting how the body changes, not just physically, but also in awareness. Once you experience a new standard of health, returning to old habits feels unnatural. Yet, it happens. I know people who began their Raw Vegan journey with enthusiasm but slowly drifted back to cooked and processed foods. The old signals, memories, and social pressures can be strong.

If that happens to you, **don't lose hope**. The beauty of the human body is that it's forgiving and always ready to heal. The moment you stop adding toxins, it begins to cleanse itself again. Remember how amazing you felt when you were living naturally; that feeling can always return.

Today, it's easier than ever to stay motivated. Online resources, social media groups, and educational videos allow you to connect with like-minded people around the world. Surrounding yourself with supportive communities can make an enormous difference when temptation or doubt appears.

If you keep faith in yourself and stay determined, you'll find your rhythm again. Every step forward counts. The rewards which are renewed energy, clearer thinking, and confidence in your body's strength, are lasting and real. You'll gain not only physical health but also the deep satisfaction of knowing that you've reclaimed control of your wellbeing and your future.

And one day, when your GP calls and asks to catch up for a coffee, your answer might be:

"Doctor, I am now a **Raw** Vegan and have found my **Ultimate Health**. I no longer drink **unhealthy beverages**! Bud I'd love to meet up and **share my secrets** with you!"

Closing Thoughts

Everything shared in this book comes from my own life journey and personal experience in pursuing what I call Ultimate Health. I've learned that nothing in this world is perfect, not even the natural lifestyle. Every path comes with challenges, but when your body runs on clean, natural fuel, those challenges become easier to handle, both physically and emotionally.

For me, this lifestyle continues to evolve. Even now, I sometimes feel the need to fine-tune it, to listen more closely to my body, to explore new foods, and to nourish my cells with the best that nature can offer. Health is not a destination; it's a lifelong relationship with your body and the natural world around you.

Much of the wisdom I've gained came from others who walked this path before me, people who shared their discoveries, insights, and experiences with honesty and generosity. I've learned from them, tested their ideas in my own life, and passed forward only what has truly worked.

Your journey, however, will be your own. Our differences in genetics, environment, culture, and access to food shape how each of us thrives. What works perfectly for one person might not be identical for another, and that's okay. What matters most is developing awareness, curiosity, and consistency.

My hope is that this book has sparked inspiration within you, encouraging you to question, explore, and discover what true health really means. Even if you're not ready to change everything right away, start with what you can. Maybe add more raw foods to your meals or remove some heavily processed, unhealthy items from your basket. Eat more fruits, fresh salads, and simple vegan dishes, or at least try going fully raw when you're unwell and see how your body responds. Small, conscious choices, one meal, one habit, one thought at a time can set you on a path to profound transformation.

May you live a long, vibrant, and fulfilling life. One where your body, mind, and spirit move in harmony, and where every moment feels rich with energy, clarity, and joy.

Amen

Enjoyed Health on Fire?

If this book lit a spark for you; helped you see your health in a new light, answered questions, or simply gave you hope; I'd be truly grateful if you could take a moment to leave an **honest, unbiased review**. Your feedback not only supports my mission to help more people reclaim their health naturally; it also helps others find this book when they need it most.

Grab the **Quick Guide to the Raw Diet + 7-Day Raw Meal Plan**; normally a $199 resource, but **Free** for all readers. Email your proof of purchase to: info@michaelzara.com.au with the subject **"Reader Bonus – Health on Fire"** and you'll receive a copy!

You can leave a quick review on

Amazon: https://www.amazon.com/dp/B0DNK3JW87

Goodreads:https://www.goodreads.com/book/show/221406164-health-on-fire

Thank you so much! — Michael Zara- Author of Health on Fire

About the Author

Michael Zara is a nutritionist, health coach, and the author of *Health on Fire*. His passion for natural healing and raw nutrition was born from his own journey of overcoming chronic health issues through a Raw Vegan lifestyle. After more than two decades of personal research, experimentation, and study, he has dedicated his life to helping others reclaim their health by understanding the body's natural needs.

Michael's formal training includes a nutrition course from *The Nutrition Institute of Australia*, which deepened his knowledge of how food impacts not only physical vitality but also emotional wellbeing and mental clarity. Beyond formal education, he has spent years reading, researching, and interviewing health professionals, naturopaths, and everyday people who have healed through natural living.

Alongside devoting himself fully to health and education, Michael has spent over 27 years as a mechanical engineer, designing and developing air conditioning systems and managing business operations across Australia. His technical background shaped his analytical approach to health; blending logic, evidence, and lived experience to uncover the principles of true wellbeing.

Today, Michael lives in Melbourne, Australia, with his wife Emma and their three children. Alongside his work in the air conditioning industry, he continues to inspire others as a health coach, guiding people toward *Ultimate Health* through education, awareness, and the power of raw, living foods.

Acknowledgement

I always appreciate and acknowledge the outstanding contributions of educators and mentors who have greatly advanced human health by following their natural paths and sharing their knowledge with others. I also want to extend a heartfelt thank you to the individuals who have helped me on my amazing journey, whom I mention below.

- With heartfelt thanks to my lovely and supportive wife, **Emma**, and to my exceptional children, whose patience and encouragement gave me the time and space to write and complete this book.

- I am deeply grateful to my wonderful **parents**, who raised me with love, integrity, and a strong respect for education. They instilled in me the importance of science and its role in understanding the world. I also extend my heartfelt thanks to my siblings, whose support has always been a guiding light, especially **my sister**, whose encouragement meant so much throughout this journey.

- **Iraj**, my soccer teammate who started the conversation about Raw eating and guided me on the path.

- **Anne Osborne** has inspired me by teaching in her book "Fruitarian, the Path to Paradise" and the helpful information she shared with me in the interviews.

- **Don Bennet**, who helped me to address my iodine and Vitamin D deficiency and shared his experiences through his helpful articles on his website, health101.org

- My guru, **Hovansian**, with his excellent book "Raw Living" which was my starting point of going fully Raw.

- My nutrition teacher, **Kassandra Kaleda**, helped me learn about nutrition and diet at The Nutrition Institute.

- My advanced nutrition teacher, **Courtney Myers**, helped me to finish my Advanced Plant-Based Diet course with the highest mark.

- **My teachers** at Box Hill Institute, who taught me about Australian culture and its wonderful community through my successful ESL course during the early stages of my arrival to Australia.

- **Doctors and dietitians** who taught me a lot about diseases, health, and medical science.

- **My friends and family** members who have supported me in this journey.

- **Jamie Pounds**, a pure, lovely person who has supported my Ultimate Health with his nutrition advice and his wonderful products of pure organic barley grass juice powders.

- **Emily LeVault**, who has edited this book.

- **Pixel Studio** which helped on designing the cover of the book.

- The businesses and companies that supplied the best Raw Vegan foods, supplements, and nutrition.

- And finally, thank you to the businesses who helped me publish this book and distribute it to society.

Credits and Sources

Sources

Organisations:

National library of medicine- USA per web address: https://www.ncbi.nlm.nih.gov/

Cancer in Australia per web addresses:

www.canceraustralia.gov.au

https://www.cancer.org.au/

Harward University USA and its medical school per web address: https://www.hsph.harvard.edu/

Proceedings of the National Academy of Sciences of the United States of America" (PNAS) per web address:

www.PNAS.org

Health Line- Evidence-based health information and advice per web address:

www.Healthline.com

Web Credits

https://frugivorebiology.com/optimal-human-foods/

https://nutrigardens.com/blogs/blog/skin-health-8-benefits-of-sunlight-the-natural-nitric-oxide-booster#:~:text=Sunlight%20as%20a%20nitric%20oxide,production%20on%20the%20skin%20surface.

https://www.outsideonline.com/health/nutrition/sunlight-may-be-next-beet-juice/

http://health101.org/

https://holisticprimarycare.net/topics/nutrition-a-lifestyle/sulfate-the-most-common-nutritional-deficiency-you-ve-never-heard

http://orthomolecular.org/resources/omns/v13n14.shtml

https://aqlivia.com/iodine

https://www.westonaprice.org/health-topics/modern-diseases/cholesterol-sulfate-deficiency-coronary-heart-disease

https://www.thenutritioninstitute.com.au/

https://www.sciencedirect.com/

https://www.frontiersin.org/

https://www.researchgate.net/

https://vegfaqs.com/essential-amino-acid-profiles-nuts/

References

Cooking and formation of oxidised materials

When food or nutrients are described as "already Oxidised," it typically means they have undergone some degree of chemical oxidation, which can alter their structure and potential for use by cells. The ability of a cell to metabolise oxidised food depends on the extent of oxidation and the type of nutrient involved.

1. Oxidised Fats

Effect: Fats can become oxidised when exposed to oxygen, heat, or light, leading to the formation of harmful compounds like lipid peroxides and free radicals.

Metabolism: oxidised fats are less efficient as an energy source and can be harmful to cells. They may contribute to cellular damage and inflammation. Cells may attempt to detoxify these oxidised compounds, but excessive intake of oxidised fats can overwhelm cellular repair mechanisms and lead to oxidative stress.

2. Oxidised Proteins

Effect: Proteins can also undergo oxidation, leading to changes in their structure and function. Oxidised proteins may form cross-links or aggregates that are difficult for cells to break down.

Metabolism: Cells have mechanisms to degrade damaged or oxidised proteins, such as through the ubiquitin-proteasome system or autophagy. However, heavily oxidised proteins may be less useful as a source of amino acids, and their accumulation can be toxic to cells.

3. Oxidised Carbohydrates

Effect: Carbohydrates are less prone to oxidation compared to fats and proteins, but when they do oxidise, it can affect their usability as an energy source.

Metabolism: Oxidised carbohydrates may be less efficient in providing energy through glycolysis and cellular respiration. However, cells can still metabolise them to some extent, depending on the degree of oxidation.

4. Vitamins and Antioxidants

Effect: Certain vitamins, particularly those with antioxidant properties (like Vitamin C and E), can become oxidised. Once oxidised, they lose their effectiveness in neutralising free radicals and may even become pro-oxidants.

Metabolism: Oxidised vitamins are generally less beneficial and may not perform their intended roles in cellular metabolism. Cells cannot easily reverse the oxidation of these nutrients.

5. General Cellular Response to Oxidised Nutrients

Cells have mechanisms to deal with oxidised molecules, such as enzymes that repair or remove damaged molecules (e.g., glutathione peroxidase, superoxide dismutase). Excessive intake of oxidised nutrients can overwhelm these protective systems, leading to oxidative stress, which is associated with various diseases, including cardiovascular diseases, cancer, and neurodegenerative disorders.

Summary

Cells can metabolise some oxidised food components, but they are less efficient and can lead to cellular damage if consumed in large amounts. Oxidised fats, proteins, and vitamins are particularly problematic, as they can contribute to oxidative stress and inflammation. Therefore, it's generally better for health to consume fresh, un-oxidised foods to support optimal cellular function.

Several studies have shown that cooking, particularly at high temperatures, can lead to the formation of oxidised materials, including oxidised fats and proteins. These oxidised compounds can form through various processes such as oxidation, Maillard reactions, and thermal degradation. Here's a brief overview of the evidence:

1. Oxidation of Fats:

- High-Temperature Cooking: Cooking methods like frying, grilling, and roasting, which involve high temperatures, can lead to the oxidation of fats, particularly unsaturated fats. This process forms lipid peroxides and other reactive oxygen species (ROS), which can degrade into potentially harmful compounds like aldehydes.

- Study Evidence: Research published in journals like *Food Chemistry* and *Journal of Agricultural and Food Chemistry* has shown that prolonged exposure to high temperatures increases the rate of lipid oxidation in cooking oils and fatty foods.

2. Protein Oxidation:

- Formation of Advanced Glycation End Products (AGEs): Cooking proteins, especially at high temperatures, can lead to the formation of oxidised proteins and AGEs. These compounds form when proteins or fats combine with sugars through a process called glycation.

- Study Evidence: Studies published in journals such as *Free Radical Biology and Medicine* and *The American Journal of Clinical Nutrition* have demonstrated that cooking methods like grilling and frying increase the concentration of AGEs and Oxidised proteins in food.

3. Oxidation of Carbohydrates:

- Maillard Reaction: This reaction between reducing sugars and amino acids during cooking, particularly under dry heat, can lead to the formation of browning and oxidised compounds.

- Study Evidence: Research has shown that the Maillard reaction, while contributing to flavour and colour, can also produce potentially harmful oxidised compounds, as documented in journals like *Critical Reviews in Food Science and Nutrition*.

4. Formation of Harmful Compounds:

- Heterocyclic Amines (HCAs) and Polycyclic Aromatic Hydrocarbons (PAHs): These are formed when meat is cooked at high temperatures, such as grilling or barbecuing. Both HCAs and PAHs are products of protein and fat oxidation and are considered potential carcinogens.

- Study Evidence: Numerous studies, including those published in *Carcinogenesis* and *Food and Chemical Toxicology*, have identified the formation of HCAs and PAHs during high-temperature cooking as a health concern.

Oxidised foods and the impact on cellular health- The information provided about the metabolism of oxidised foods and the impact on cellular health is based on well-established biochemical and nutritional principles. While the explanation is drawn from general scientific knowledge, I can summarise key points and provide references to support the discussion.

Key Concepts and References

Oxidised Fats:

Impact on Health: Oxidised fats, particularly those containing lipid peroxides, can lead to oxidative stress and inflammation. These compounds are known to be harmful and contribute to various diseases, including atherosclerosis.

References:

Halliwell, B., & Gutteridge, J. M. C. (2015). Free Radicals in Biology and Medicine (5th ed.). Oxford University Press.

Kanner, J. (2007). Dietary advanced lipid oxidation end products are risk factors to human health. Molecular Nutrition & Food Research, 51(9), 1094-1101.

Oxidised Proteins:

Cellular Handling: Oxidised proteins can be recognised and degraded by cellular mechanisms like the ubiquitin-proteasome system or autophagy. Accumulation of oxidised proteins is linked to aging and various diseases.

References:

Stadtman, E. R. (2006). Protein oxidation and aging. Free Radical Research, 40(12), 1250-1258.

Levine, R. L., & Stadtman, E. R. (2001). Oxidative modification of proteins during aging. Experimental Gerontology, 36(9), 1495-1502.

Oxidised Carbohydrates:

Metabolic Impact: While carbohydrates are less prone to oxidation, the presence of oxidised sugars (e.g., advanced glycation end products) can negatively affect cellular function and contribute to conditions like diabetes.

References:

Ramasamy, R., Vannucci, S. J., Yan, S. S., Herold, K., Yan, S. F., & Schmidt, A. M. (2005). Advanced glycation end products and RAGE: a common thread in aging, diabetes, neurodegeneration, and inflammation. Glycobiology, 15(7), 16R-28R.

Oxidised Vitamins and Antioxidants:

Nutritional Role: Antioxidant vitamins, such as Vitamin C and E, lose their protective effects when oxidised. This can diminish their role in preventing oxidative damage to cells.

References:

Traber, M. G., & Atkinson, J. (2007). Vitamin E, antioxidant and nothing more. Free Radical Biology and Medicine, 43(1), 4-15.

Carr, A. C., & Frei, B. (1999). Toward a new recommended dietary allowance for vitamin C based on antioxidant and health effects in humans. The American Journal of Clinical Nutrition, 69(6), 1086-1107.

General Cellular Response to Oxidative Stress:

Protective Mechanisms: Cells use enzymes like glutathione peroxidase and superoxide dismutase to neutralise oxidative damage. However, excessive oxidative stress can overwhelm these systems, leading to cell damage and disease.

References:

Sies, H. (1997). Oxidative stress: oxidants and antioxidants. Experimental Physiology, 82(2), 291-295.

Droge, W. (2002). Free radicals in the physiological control of cell function. Physiological Reviews, 82(1), 47-95.

Lipid Oxidation and Free Radical Formation:

Study: A study published in Food Chemistry (2016) investigated lipid oxidation in various cooking oils when exposed to high temperatures.

Findings: The researchers found that heating oils, especially at high temperatures like those used in frying, leads to the formation of lipid peroxides and free radicals. These compounds are responsible for oxidative stress, which can contribute to various health issues when consumed.

Effects of Cooking on Meat

Study: Research published in the Journal of Agricultural and Food Chemistry (2008) examined the formation of free radicals in different types of meat (beef, chicken, pork) during cooking.

Findings: The study showed that cooking methods such as grilling, broiling, and frying produced more free radicals in meat compared to boiling or steaming.

The formation of free radicals was linked to the oxidation of fats and the **Maillard** reaction (a chemical reaction between amino acids and sugars that gives browned food its distinctive flavor).

Antioxidant Degradation in Vegetables:

Study: A study in the Journal of Food Science (2009) analysed the effect of various cooking methods on the antioxidant content and free radical scavenging ability of vegetables.

Findings: High-temperature cooking methods, like frying and roasting, significantly reduced the levels of antioxidants such as vitamin C and phenolic compounds in vegetables. The loss of these antioxidants was associated with an increased potential for free radical formation.

Formation of Reactive Oxygen Species (ROS) in Fried Foods:

Study: A paper in Food and Chemical Toxicology (2010) investigated the formation of reactive oxygen species (ROS) during the frying process.

Findings: The research demonstrated that frying oils, especially after repeated use, produced significant amounts of ROS, which are a type of free radical. These ROS were shown to increase oxidative stress in the body when the fried foods were consumed.

Cooking Oil Stability and Free Radical Formation:

Study: Research published in Food Research International (2017) focused on the stability of various cooking oils under heat and their tendency to form free radicals.

Findings: The study found that oils with a high content of unsaturated fats (like sunflower and corn oil) were more prone to oxidation and free radical formation when heated, especially at high temperatures. Saturated fats, like those in coconut oil, were more stable under heat but still produced free radicals to some extent.

Antioxidant Loss: The degradation of antioxidants like vitamins C and E during cooking can reduce the food's ability to neutralise free radicals, indirectly contributing to oxidative stress.

Free radicals in biology and medicine" (Halliwell and Gutteridge, 2007) is a widely cited book that explores the role of free radicals in various diseases, including CVD and cancer. Review articles and meta-analyses, such as "Oxidative stress in atherosclerosis: The role of oxidised LDL and noxious radicals" (American Journal of Physiology, 1993), provide comprehensive insights into the role of oxidative stress in cardiovascular diseases.

Impact of nutrition on cellular health:

Nutrient Availability and Cell Function: Vitamin and Mineral Deficiencies: Studies have examined how deficiencies in vitamins (e.g., B vitamins, vitamin D) and minerals (e.g., zinc, magnesium) can affect cell function and division. For example:

"Micronutrients and DNA Damage: The Role of Vitamins in the Prevention of Cellular Damage and Cancer" (Nutrients, 2013).

"The Role of Zinc in Cellular Homeostasis and Its Impact on Cellular Health" (Nutrients, 2016).

Impact of Diet on Cellular Health: Inflammation and Oxidative Stress: Research exploring how diets high in sugar and unhealthy fats contribute to inflammation and oxidative stress includes:

"Dietary Sugar and Cardiovascular Disease Risk: A Review of the Evidence" (Nutrients, 2017).

"Dietary Fats and Health: Dietary Recommendations in the Context of Scientific Evidence" (Nutrients, 2018).

Effects of Diet on Cancer Cells: Cancer Metabolism: Research on how sugar and processed foods impact cancer cells:

"The Warburg Effect: A Metabolic Phenomenon in Cancer" (Journal of Clinical Investigation, 2006).

"Impact of High Sugar Consumption on Cancer Risk: Systematic Review and Meta-Analysis" (International Journal of Cancer, 2016).

Cellular Aging and Diet: Diet and Cellular Aging: Studies on how diet impacts cellular aging and health:

"Nutritional Influences on Cellular Aging and Longevity" (Nutrients, 2016).

"The Role of Antioxidants in Cellular Aging and Health" (Free Radical Biology and Medicine, 2018).

Enzymes - A comprehensive review by Bengmark (2012) discusses the changes in digestive enzyme production and function with aging. The review highlights how reduced enzyme levels can lead to diminished digestive efficiency and nutrient absorption. A study by Morley and colleagues (1997) examined changes in pancreatic function with age. The research demonstrated a reduction in pancreatic enzyme output, impacting fat digestion and absorption.

Gut neurons - Approximately 90-95% of the body's serotonin is found in the gastrointestinal tract, where it is synthesised and stored by enterochromaffin cells. The book "The Second Brain" by Michael D. Gershon, a pioneer in the study of the ENS, explores the significance of the neurons in the gut and their relationship to overall health.

Animal products and health - Sacks et al. (2017) conducted a comprehensive review on dietary fats and cardiovascular disease. The study highlighted that saturated fats, primarily found in animal products, are associated with increased levels of LDL cholesterol, a major risk factor for cardiovascular disease. Reference: Sacks, F. M., Lichtenstein, A. H., Wu, J. H., Appel, L. J., Creager, M. A., Kris-Etherton, P. M., ... & Van Horn, L. V. (2017). Dietary Fats and Cardiovascular Disease: A Presidential Advisory From the American Heart Association. Circulation, 136(3), e1-e23.

The World Health Organization's International Agency for Research on Cancer (IARC) classified processed meat as a Group 1 carcinogen and red meat as a Group 2A carcinogen based on sufficient evidence linking consumption to colorectal cancer. Reference: Bouvard, V., Loomis, D., Guyton, K. Z., Grosse, Y., Ghissassi, F. E., Benbrahim-Tallaa, L., ... &

Straif, K. (2015). Carcinogenicity of consumption of red and processed meat. The Lancet Oncology, 16(16), 1599-1600.

Diabetes, Overall Mortality, Inflammation and **Gut Health.**

Obesity related diseases- Framingham Heart Study- This long-term, ongoing cardiovascular cohort study has been instrumental in identifying the links between obesity and various cardiovascular diseases, including coronary heart disease, hypertension, and stroke.

Research published in journals like The Lancet and Diabetes Care has consistently demonstrated the strong association between obesity and the development of type 2 diabetes. The presence of excess body fat, particularly visceral fat, has been linked to insulin resistance and impaired glucose metabolism.

The WHO has extensively documented the health risks associated with obesity, highlighting its role in increasing the risk of cardiovascular diseases, diabetes, musculoskeletal disorders like osteoarthritis, and certain cancers.

Global warming- The Food and Agriculture Organization (FAO) of the United Nations published a comprehensive report titled "Livestock's Long Shadow," which discusses the environmental impact of livestock production, including methane emissions from enteric fermentation in ruminants like cows. Reference: Saunois, M., Stavert, A. R., Poulter, B., Bousquet, P., Canadell, J. G., Jackson, R. B., ... & Zickfeld, K. (2020). The Global Methane Budget 2000–2017. Earth System Science Data, 12(3), 1561-1623.

Animal products related diseases- Studies published in journals like The New England Journal of Medicine and The Lancet have demonstrated that diets high in saturated fats and cholesterol, often found in red and processed meats, can increase LDL cholesterol levels. Elevated LDL cholesterol is a known risk factor for atherosclerosis and coronary heart disease.

The International Agency for Research on Cancer (IARC), part of the World Health Organization, has classified processed meat as a Group 1 carcinogen, meaning it has sufficient evidence of causing cancer in humans, particularly colorectal cancer.

A documentary called "**What the Health**" on Netflix worth watching.

Uric Acid- Research published in Diabetes Care found that hyperuricemia (elevated uric acid) was a predictor of incident type 2 diabetes. The proposed mechanisms include the role of uric acid in promoting insulin resistance and impairing endothelial function.

Research published in Hypertension and other journals suggests that uric acid may contribute to high blood pressure by reducing nitric oxide production, leading to vasoconstriction, and by stimulating the renin-angiotensin system, which regulates blood pressure. High uric acid levels have also been associated with Non-Alcoholic Fatty Liver Disease (NAFLD). Studies, including those in Hepatology, have demonstrated that hyperuricemia is often present in patients with NAFLD and may be involved in the pathogenesis of the disease. Uric acid can promote oxidative stress and inflammation in the liver, contributing to the accumulation of fat and the progression of liver damage.

The mechanisms by which uric acid contributes to these conditions include the promotion of oxidative stress, inflammation, endothelial dysfunction, and insulin resistance. Uric acid can act as a pro-oxidant, leading to oxidative damage in tissues and organs, which may exacerbate metabolic dysfunction.

Our Ancestors- Fossils of early human ancestors, such as Australopithecus afarensis (e.g., the famous "Lucy" specimen), Homo habilis, and Homo erectus, have been found in East Africa, particularly in the Great Rift Valley, which provides strong evidence that early hominins lived in these regions.

Stone tools and other artifacts found in Africa date back to the earliest known human cultures, further supporting the idea that modern humans originated in Africa.

References:

"**The Cradle of Humankind**" by Donald Johanson and Blake Edgar.

"**The Origins of Modern Humans**" by Fred H. Smith and James C. Ahern

"**Out of Africa Again and Again**" by Chris Stringer and Robin McKie

Protein RDI- The Institute of Medicine (IOM)provides recommended dietary allowances (RDAs) for protein intake. For an average adult, the RDA is about 0.8 grams of protein per kilogram of body weight per day. For a 70 kg adult, this equals approximately 56 grams of protein per day. These recommendations are designed to meet the nutritional needs of nearly all (97-98%) healthy individuals.

Studies on protein utilisation, such as those examining the Protein Digestibility Corrected Amino Acid Score (PDCAAS) or the Digestible Indispensable Amino Acid Score (DIAAS), explore how efficiently the body can use different proteins. These studies sometimes suggest lower thresholds for essential amino acids intake, especially when consuming highly bioavailable protein sources.

Sugar and Cancer Cells- Studies, such as those published in Cancer Epidemiology, Biomarkers & Prevention, have linked high levels of insulin and IGF-1 with an increased risk of cancers, including breast and colorectal cancer. The concept originates from the work of Otto Warburg in the 1920s, who observed that cancer cells often exhibit high rates of glycolysis followed by lactic acid fermentation, even under normal oxygen conditions. This was contrary to the typical energy production pathway in healthy cells, which rely more on oxidative phosphorylation.

Modern studies, such as those published in Nature Reviews Cancer and Cell Metabolism, have expanded on Warburg's findings, exploring the metabolic adaptations in cancer cells that allow them to thrive in various environments, including nutrient-limited conditions.

Fruits and Diabetes- Nurses' Health Study and Health Professionals Follow-Up Study: These large, long-term cohort studies have provided significant evidence on the relationship between fruit consumption and diabetes risk.

A study published in BMJ (a weekly peer-reviewed medical journal, published by BMJ Group, which in turn is wholly-owned by the British Medical Association) in 2013 analysed data from these cohorts and found that higher intake of specific whole fruits, particularly blueberries, grapes, and apples, was associated with a reduced risk of type 2 diabetes.

Meta-Analysis on Fruit Consumption: A meta-analysis published in Diabetes Care in 2014 examined multiple prospective cohort studies and found that a higher intake of whole fruits was associated with a lower risk of type 2 diabetes. The study emphasised that the protective effect was particularly strong for berries, apples, and citrus fruits.

Fruits are also rich in antioxidants and phytochemicals, such as polyphenols, which have anti-inflammatory and insulin-sensitising properties. Research in Nutrition & Diabetes and The Journal of Nutrition has shown that these compounds can improve insulin sensitivity and reduce oxidative stress, which are important factors in diabetes prevention.

Omega-3 VS Omega-6- Evolutionary Diets: Research published in Biomedicine & Pharmacotherapy by Artemis Simopoulos has explored the evolutionary aspects of fatty acid intake, suggesting that the diet of early humans was closer to a 1:1 ratio of Omega-6 to Omega-3 fatty acids. This balance is thought to have played a role in reducing inflammation and chronic diseases.

A review article in The American Journal of Clinical Nutrition highlights how Omega-6 fatty acids, predominantly linoleic acid, can be converted into arachidonic acid, a precursor for pro-inflammatory eicosanoids. In contrast, Omega-3 fatty acids, such as EPA and DHA, are precursors to anti-inflammatory eicosanoids.

An imbalance, with a high Omega-6 to Omega-3 ratio, can promote inflammation and is associated with an increased risk of chronic diseases, including cardiovascular disease, cancer, and autoimmune disorders.

A paper published by Artemis P. Simopoulos in the journal Biomedicine & Pharmacotherapy titled "The importance of the ratio of omega-6/omega-3 essential fatty acids" discusses how modern dietary practices have led to Omega-6/Omega-3 ratios ranging from 10:1 to 20:1 in some Western diets, including the United States.

Another study by Hibbeln et al., published in The American Journal of Clinical Nutrition (2006), also highlighted similar findings, reporting that Omega-6 to Omega-3 ratios in the U.S. could range from 10:1 to 17:1.

Vitamin C Loss- Studies on the degradation of Vitamin C in foods, such as those published in Food Chemistry and Journal of Agricultural and Food Chemistry, have documented the impact of food preparation methods on the nutrient's stability. These studies often find that exposure to air and light can result in significant losses of Vitamin C.

Dairy and Osteoporosis- Some epidemiological data have indicated that countries with high dairy consumption, such as the United States and Scandinavian countries, also report higher rates of osteoporosis and hip fractures. This paradox has been noted in studies and reviews, including those published in The Journal of Nutrition and Osteoporosis International.

Skin Cancers and Sunscreens- Data from various countries, including the United States, Australia, and parts of Europe, indicate that the incidence of skin cancer, particularly melanoma, has been rising. This trend is documented in research published in journals such as JAMA Dermatology and Cancer Epidemiology, Biomarkers & Prevention.

These studies often highlight that the increase in skin cancer rates has occurred despite the growing availability and use of sunscreens.

There is concern that certain nanoparticles, particularly titanium dioxide, may be photoreactive, meaning they can produce reactive oxygen species (ROS) when exposed to UV light. ROS are highly reactive molecules that can damage cellular structures, including DNA, potentially leading to skin aging and cancer. Research in Environmental Health Perspectives and Nanotoxicology has investigated the phototoxicity of these nanoparticles, particularly when they are not coated with protective layers.

Chronic Stress- The concept of allostatic load refers to the cumulative burden of chronic stress and the body's efforts to maintain stability (homeostasis) through physiological adaptation. Research published in Psychosomatic Medicine and Annual Review of Public Health has shown that high allostatic load is associated with numerous health problems, including cardiovascular disease, obesity, diabetes, and immune system dysfunction.

Studies such as those in Circulation and The Lancet have demonstrated that stress-related hormones like cortisol and adrenaline can lead to long-term increases in blood pressure and other cardiovascular risk factors.

Exercise and Lymph system- General research on exercise physiology shows that physical activity enhances lymphatic circulation, which can help with detoxification, immune function, and fluid balance.

Techniques like manual lymphatic drainage, rebound exercises (like using a trampoline), and even simple activities like walking or stretching are known to stimulate lymph flow.

Copyright

Glossary

ALS stands for **A**myotrophic **L**ateral **S**clerosis, also known as Lou Gehrig's disease. It is a progressive neurodegenerative disease that affects nerve cells in the brain and the spinal cord. Over time, ALS leads to the degeneration of motor neurons, which are responsible for controlling voluntary muscle movements. As the disease progresses, individuals with ALS may experience muscle weakness, twitching, stiffness, and eventually paralysis.

Alzheimer's disease is a progressive neurodegenerative disorder that primarily affects memory, thinking, and behavior. It is the most common cause of dementia, accounting for 60-80% of dementia cases. Alzheimer's disease gradually destroys brain cells, leading to a decline in cognitive functions and the ability to carry out daily activities. The condition typically affects older adults, although it can occur in younger people in rare cases (early-onset Alzheimer's).

Anemia is a medical condition characterised by a deficiency in the number or quality of red blood cells (RBCs) or hemoglobin in the blood. Hemoglobin is the protein in red blood cells that carries oxygen from the lungs to the rest of the body. When you have anemia, your body doesn't get enough oxygen-rich blood, leading to symptoms like fatigue, weakness, shortness of breath, and pale skin. Diagnosis typically involves blood tests to measure hemoglobin levels, red blood cell count, and other parameters. Treatment depends on the type and cause of anemia and may include dietary changes, supplements (iron, vitamin B12, folate), medications, or procedures like blood transfusions or bone marrow transplants in severe cases.

Antihistamines are a class of drugs that counteract the effects of histamine, a substance in the body that is released during allergic reactions. They are commonly used to treat symptoms of allergies, such as sneezing, itching, watery eyes, and runny nose. Antihistamines can also be used to treat other conditions, such as motion sickness, insomnia, and certain symptoms of the common cold.

Arthritis (Rheumatoid arthritis (RA)) is a general term that refers to a group of more than 100 different types of inflammatory joint disorders. These conditions cause inflammation, pain, and stiffness in the affected joints, which can lead to reduced range of motion and functional impairment. Arthritis can affect people of all ages, including children, but it is more common in older adults.

Asthma is a chronic respiratory condition that affects the airways in the lungs. It causes the airways to become inflamed, narrow, and produce extra mucus, leading to breathing difficulties. The severity of asthma symptoms can vary widely, from mild and infrequent to severe and persistent.

Autophagy (from Greek, meaning "self-eating") is the body's natural process of cleaning out damaged or unnecessary cells. (See Glossary) and recycling their components to create new, healthy ones. It's like an internal repair and renewal system.

Some studies suggest that fasting; including dry fasting; may activate autophagy, the body's natural cellular repair and recycling process. However, this link is not yet fully proven or accepted by mainstream medical science, especially regarding dry fasting in humans. Most research supporting autophagy comes from animal or laboratory studies, so more evidence is needed before firm conclusions can be made.

Beta Cells in the Pancreas are one of the several types of cells found within the islets of Langerhans. They are crucial for the endocrine function of the pancreas because they produce and secrete **insulin**, a hormone that regulates blood glucose (sugar) levels.

Cardiovascular diseases (CVD) refer to a group of disorders affecting the heart and blood vessels. These conditions are the leading cause of death globally and can result from a variety of factors, including lifestyle, genetics, and other underlying health conditions.

Common types of cardiovascular diseases include:

1. **Coronary Artery Disease (CAD):** This is the most common type of CVD and occurs when the blood vessels that supply

blood to the heart become narrowed or blocked due to the buildup of plaque (atherosclerosis). This can lead to chest pain (angina), heart attacks, or other serious complications.

2. **Heart Attack (Myocardial Infarction):** A heart attack occurs when a blood clot blocks the flow of blood to a part of the heart muscle, causing damage or death to the tissue. It's often a result of coronary artery disease.

3. **Stroke:** A stroke occurs when the blood supply to part of the brain is interrupted or reduced, causing brain cells to die.

   It can be due to a blocked artery (ischemic stroke) or a burst blood vessel (haemorrhagic stroke).

4. **Heart Failure:** This condition occurs when the heart is unable to pump blood effectively, leading to symptoms such as shortness of breath, fatigue, and fluid retention. Heart failure can result from various CVDs, including CAD and hypertension.

5. **Arrhythmias:** These are irregular heartbeats that can be too fast, too slow, or erratic. While some arrhythmias are harmless, others can be life-threatening and may require medical intervention.

6. **Hypertension (High Blood Pressure):** Chronic high blood pressure can damage the heart and blood vessels, increasing the risk of other cardiovascular diseases, such as heart attack, stroke, and heart failure.

7. **Peripheral Artery Disease (PAD):** This condition occurs when the arteries that supply blood to the limbs (usually the legs) become narrowed or blocked, leading to pain, cramping, and, in severe cases, tissue damage.

8. **Congenital Heart Defects:** These are structural abnormalities of the heart that are present from birth. They can affect the heart's function and may require surgical or medical treatment.

Catalyst is a substance that speeds up a chemical reaction without being consumed or permanently altered in the process. Catalysts work by lowering the activation energy required for a reaction to occur, allowing the reaction to proceed more quickly or at a lower temperature. They are crucial in many industrial and biological processes. In human biology, catalysts are typically enzymes. Enzymes are proteins that speed up biochemical reactions in the body without being consumed in the process. They work by lowering the activation energy required for a reaction, making it easier for the reaction to occur.

Cirrhosis is a more advanced and severe stage of liver disease characterised by the replacement of healthy liver tissue with scar tissue (fibrosis). This scarring disrupts the normal structure and function of the liver, leading to progressive liver damage and impaired liver function.

Endometriosis is a chronic medical condition where tissue similar to the lining inside the uterus, called the endometrium, grows outside the uterus. This abnormal growth can occur on the ovaries, fallopian tubes, the outer surface of the uterus, and other organs within the pelvis. In rare cases, it can spread beyond the pelvic region.

Enzymes are proteins that speed up biochemical reactions necessary for life. Enzymes are crucial for numerous processes, including digestion, metabolism, DNA replication, and more.

Fatty liver or hepatic steatosis is a condition where excess fat builds up in the liver cells. It's often considered an early stage of liver disease and can progress if left untreated.

There are two types of Fatty Liver:

1. **Non-Alcoholic Fatty Liver Disease (NAFLD):** This is the most common form and is not directly related to alcohol consumption. It is often associated with obesity, insulin resistance, high blood sugar, and high levels of fats in the blood (e.g., triglycerides). NAFLD can progress to a more severe

condition known as non-alcoholic steatohepatitis (NASH), which involves inflammation and liver damage.

2. **Alcoholic Fatty Liver Disease:** This form is caused by excessive alcohol consumption. The liver processes alcohol, but excessive intake can overwhelm the liver, leading to fat accumulation. If drinking continues, it can lead to more severe liver damage.

Fibromyalgia is a chronic disorder characterised by widespread musculoskeletal pain, fatigue, and tenderness in localised areas of the body. It affects how the brain processes pain signals, amplifying painful sensations.

Hyponatremia is a condition characterised by an abnormally low level of sodium in the blood. Sodium is an essential electrolyte that helps regulate water balance in and around cells, and it's crucial for nerve and muscle function. Hyponatremia can occur due to various factors however it can happen mainly by excessive water intake which drinking too much water can dilute the sodium in the blood.

Metabolism refers to the complex set of chemical reactions that occur within living organisms to maintain life. These reactions are responsible for converting the food we eat into energy that the body needs to function, as well as for building and repairing tissues, and managing waste products.

Metabolism is typically divided into two main categories:

1. **Catabolism:** This is the process of breaking down molecules to produce energy. For example, during digestion, the body breaks down carbohydrates, fats, and proteins from food into smaller molecules like glucose, fatty acids, and amino acids. These molecules are then used to produce energy, primarily in the form of adenosine triphosphate (ATP), which powers various cellular processes.

2. **Anabolism:** This is the process of building up or synthesising complex molecules from simpler ones. Anabolism uses the

energy produced during catabolism to construct and repair tissues, synthesise hormones, and carry out other vital functions. For example, the body uses amino acids to build proteins, which are essential for muscle growth and repair.

MS - Multiple **S**clerosis is a chronic autoimmune disease that affects the central nervous system (CNS), which includes the brain and spinal cord. In MS, the immune system mistakenly attacks the protective sheath (myelin) covering the nerve fibers, causing inflammation and damage. This disrupts the normal flow of electrical impulses along the nerves, leading to a wide range of neurological symptoms.

Osteoporosis is a medical condition characterised by weakened bones, making them more fragile and susceptible to fractures. It occurs when the creation of new bone doesn't keep up with the removal of old bone, leading to decreased bone density and mass. Osteoporosis is a significant health concern, especially for older adults, and early detection and prevention are key to reducing the risk of fractures and maintaining a healthy quality of life.

Oxidation is a chemical process in which a substance loses electrons. This typically occurs when a substance reacts with oxygen, but it can happen in other ways as well. Oxidation is commonly associated with the rusting of metals, the browning of fruits, and even the process of burning. In broader terms, it refers to any reaction where the state of a molecule, atom, or ion changes, usually by losing electrons to oxygen. In biology pro-oxidants facilitate this process, leading to the production of ROS, such as superoxide anions (O_2^-), hydrogen peroxide (H_2O_2), and hydroxyl radicals ($OH\cdot$).

Panadol is a brand name for the drug paracetamol, which is also known as acetaminophen in some countries. It is commonly used as an over-the-counter medication to relieve pain and reduce fever.

Pancreas is a gland located in the abdomen, behind the stomach, and it plays a vital role in both the digestive and endocrine systems. It has two primary functions: producing digestive enzymes and regulating blood sugar levels.

Functions of the Pancreas are:

1. **Exocrine Function:** The pancreas produces digestive enzymes that help break down carbohydrates, proteins, and fats in the small intestine. These enzymes are released into the small intestine through a network of ducts. The pancreas also secretes bicarbonate to neutralise stomach acid in the small intestine.

2. **Endocrine Function:** The pancreas contains clusters of cells known as the islets of Langerhans, which are responsible for producing hormones that regulate blood sugar levels.

pH- Potential of Hydrogen, referred to as acidity or alkalinity in chemistry. pH below 7 shows the acidity of a substance, while over 7 shows it is alkaline, and 7 means it is neutral.

Pro-oxidants are substances or agents that promote oxidation, leading to the generation of Reactive Oxygen Species (ROS) and free radicals. These reactive molecules can cause damage to cells, proteins, lipids, and DNA, contributing to oxidative stress and various diseases.

Psoriasis is a chronic autoimmune skin condition that causes the rapid buildup of skin cells, leading to the formation of thick, red, scaly patches on the skin. These patches, known as plaques, can be itchy, painful, and sometimes crack or bleed. Psoriasis is a long-lasting (chronic) disease with periods of flare-ups and remission.

Rickets is a medical condition that affects bone development in children, leading to soft and weakened bones. It is primarily caused by a deficiency of vitamin D, calcium, or phosphate, which are essential nutrients for healthy bone formation. Vitamin D is crucial because it helps the body absorb calcium and phosphate from the diet. Without sufficient vitamin D, the body cannot properly regulate these minerals, leading to weak and soft bones. This can result in skeletal deformities, such as bowed legs or thickened wrists and ankles, and in severe cases, it can cause delays in growth and development.

Shingles, also known as herpes zoster, is a viral infection that causes a painful rash. It is caused by the varicella-zoster virus, the same virus responsible for chickenpox. After a person recovers from chickenpox, the virus remains dormant in the body's nerve tissues. Years later, the virus can reactivate as shingles, typically in adults or older individuals, particularly those with weakened immune systems.

Stroke, also known as a cerebrovascular accident (CVA), is a serious condition that occurs when the blood supply to part of the brain is interrupted or reduced. This deprives brain tissue of oxygen and nutrients, leading to the death of brain cells within minutes.

Type 2 diabetes is a chronic condition that affects the way the body processes blood sugar (glucose). It's characterised by insulin resistance, where the body's cells do not respond properly to insulin, a hormone produced by the pancreas that regulates blood sugar levels. Over time, the pancreas may not produce enough insulin to maintain normal blood glucose levels.

Typical Western Diet (T.W.D.) which comprises of fresh and cooked food. Typical Western Diet- which is widely accepted by many people in Europe, America, and Australia as a food pyramid and model for human nutrition. This food pyramid, which includes cooked foods, is also accepted by many people around the globe. This includes bread, cereal, rice, pasta, and potatoes; some fruits and vegetables; meat, poultry, dairy, eggs, fish; and finally, some sweets like chocolate and cakes.

www.ingramcontent.com/pod-product-compliance
Lightning Source LLC
Chambersburg PA
CBHW031118020426
42333CB00012B/133